THE
MACROBIOTIC
WAY

THE MACROBIOTIC WAY

The Complete Macrobiotic Lifestyle Book

THIRD EDITION

MICHIO KUSHI
with STEVEN BLAUER

AVERY
a member of
Penguin Group (USA) Inc.

a member of
Penguin Group (USA) Inc.
375 Hudson Street
New York, NY 10014
www.penguin.com

Library of Congress Cataloging-in-Publication Data

Kushi, Michio.
The macrobiotic way : the complete macrobiotic lifestyle book / Michio Kushi, with
Stephen Blauer.—3rd ed.
p. cm.
Previously published with subtitle: The complete macrobiotic diet & exercise book.
Includes bibliographical references and index.
ISBN 1-58333-180-8
1. Macrobiotic diet.   2. Exercise.   3. Health.   I. Blauer, Stephen.   II. Title.
RM235.K873 2004   2003061756
613.2'64—dc22

Printed in the United States of America
20 19 18 17 16 15 14 13

I dedicate this work to the memories of
my wife and daughter, Aveline and Lily,
and to all my wonderful children.
Further, I thank George and Lima Ohsawa,
and the millions of people worldwide
who share our dream of world peace
and happiness for everyone.

CONTENTS

THE
MACROBIOTIC
WAY

Preface

The earliest recorded use of the term *macrobiotics* is found in the writings of Hippocrates, the father of Western Medicine. In his essay "Airs, Waters, and Places," Hippocrates introduced the word to describe people who were healthy and long-lived. Translated from the Greek, *macro* means "large" or "great," and *bios* signifies "life." Herodotus, Aristotle, Galen, and other classical writers used the term macrobiotics to describe a lifestyle, including a simple balanced diet that promoted health and longevity.

In the late eighteenth century, the German physician and philosopher Christopher W. Hufeland renewed interest in the term. His influential book on diet and health was entitled *Macrobiotics, or The Art of Prolonging Life*.

Nearly a century later, the term *macrobiotics* experienced another revival, this time originating in Japan. Two educators, Sagen Ishizuka, M.D., and Yukikazu Sakurazawa, cured themselves of serious illnesses by adopting a simple diet of brown rice, miso soup, sea vegetables, and other traditional foods. They spent many years studying and integrating traditional Oriental medicine and Eastern philosophy with Judeo-Christian teachings and holistic perspectives in modern science and medicine. Sakurazawa went to Paris in the 1920s. Later, he adopted the name George Ohsawa and applied the term *macrobiotics* to his teachings.

From the time of his illness until his death at the age of seventy-four, Ohsawa devoted himself to defining macrobiotics as it applies to modern living. He did much to spread information about the macrobiotic lifestyle, visiting more than thirty countries, giving more than 7,000 lectures, and publishing more than three hundred books.

Ohsawa had many students, among them Michio Kushi, the author of this book. Kushi was born in 1926 and graduated from Tokyo University with a degree in international law before coming to the United States in 1949. While completing further studies at Columbia University in New York, he also began teaching the macrobiotic approach to diet and health as the areas to achieve world peace. Kushi enjoyed sharing his knowledge of macrobiotics and natural health with others so much that he made it his life's work.

When Kushi began teaching macrobiotics, he met many people who were eager to learn, but were unaccustomed to eating simple whole foods. He saw that there was a need to adapt the macrobiotic diet to modern tastes while retaining its integrity. Over the years, Kushi has traveled extensively, lecturing and teaching the macrobiotic way to groups around the world.

Macrobiotics advocates the use of traditional foods such as whole grains, beans, and locally grown vegetables as the primary sources of food energy and nutrition. In addition, the diet includes nutritious soyfoods, which have been used in Asia for hundreds of years, and mineral-rich foods from the ocean—sea vegetables and certain types of fish. In the macrobiotic diet, moderate amounts of white-meat fish and shellfish are often substituted for the red meat and poultry that are common elements of the typical Western diet. Sea salt and natural grain sweeteners such as rice syrup and barley malt replace the refined salt and sugar that currently play a major role in modern fare.

When Michio Kushi first accepted the challenge of helping people shift to a more healthful way of eating and living, he had trouble finding many of the wholesome foods that he recommended. So, with his late wife, Aveline, he started a natural foods business to fill the need. Later to be called Erewhon Foods, this small enterprise developed into a $17 million business specializing in macrobiotic and natural foods. After acquiring the nearly 100-year-old U.S. Mills, the company adopted U.S. Mills as its name, and Erewhon remains as a brand name.

To research and popularize the macrobiotic approach, Michio and Aveline Kushi founded the East-West Foundation and the Kushi Institute (of which their son Phiya is now executive director), both nonprofit educational organizations; the *East West Journal,* a monthly magazine that reached a worldwide circulation of more than 75,000 copies; and several macrobiotic restaurants. The Kushis had five children and five grandchildren.

Michio and Aveline Kushi wrote many books on macrobiotics, including *The Book of Macrobiotics; The Book of Do-In: Exercise for Physical and Spiritual Development; The Cancer Prevention Diet; Your Face Never Lies: An Introduction to Oriental Diagnosis; The Macrobiotic Approach to Cancer; Natural Healing Through Macrobiotics; How to Cook with Miso; The Changing Seasons Macrobiotic Cookbook;* and *Macrobiotic Pregnancy and Care of the Newborn.* Michio Kushi is also the author of a series of books, Teachings of Michio Kushi.

I came to know Michio and Aveline Kushi well—both extraordinary people with endless reserves of energy, patience, and compassion for others. As a scholar, philosopher, writer, and teacher, Michio Kushi is often busy from early in the morning until after midnight. Whether he is greeting individuals for counseling sessions, discussing plans for the further development and growth of the macrobiotic way, attending a session of the macrobiotic scientific committee, giving a seminar for medical and health-care professionals, or just talking about life with a friend, Kushi is always actively sharing his boundless enthusiasm for living and his ability to view life's problems with gentle good humor.

This book is the result of my desire to understand Michio Kushi's macrobiotic approach to diet and health and to explain it in simple terms to a general audience. Michio Kushi is the author of this book inasmuch as its contents are derived from discussions with him. In addition, material from his lectures, published books, and articles has been drawn upon.

Both Michio and I are indebted to our families and friends for their valuable assistance in preparing this book. We would especially like to thank Aveline Kushi and Wendy Esko for helping to develop the recipes and cooking sections, with the assistance of Karen Williamson, Caroline Heindenry, and Colleen Blauer. Special thanks also go to Lawrence Haruo Kushi of the Harvard School of Public Health, to Phillip Kushi and Ed Esko of the East West Foundation, to Bill Tara of the Kushi Institute, and to Lenny Jacobs, Linda Roszak, and Mark Mayell of the *East West Journal,* for reviewing the style, tone, accuracy, and clarity of the other sections of the book.

My greatest hope is that the spirit of sharing and cooperation, through which this book became a reality, will somehow touch the lives of its readers. For in giving is to be found abundance, peace, and happiness.

Stephen Blauer
Boston

Introduction

Macrobiotics is a way of eating and living that has been practiced for thousands of years by many people around the world. It stems from an intuitive understanding of the orderliness of nature. Modern macrobiotic philosophy focuses on offering a way of living that closes the widening gap between humans and the natural world. Macrobiotic theory suggests that sickness and unhappiness are nature's way of urging us to adopt a proper diet and way of life, and that these troubles are unnecessary when we live in harmony with our environment. The macrobiotic diet is based on whole grains and traditional foods in harmony with the seasons.

As we have become somewhat removed from the natural elements, we have lost much that is valuable. We can learn a great deal from cultures such as those of the Hunzakut people, of a region now in northeast Pakistan; the Vilcabambans, who live high in the South American Andes; and the Abkhasians, who reside in an area of the former Soviet republic of Georgia located between southern Russia and the Black Sea. One characteristic shared by these cultures is that the people often live in continuous close contact with nature. They are also vitally healthy and very active physically, many beyond their hundredth birthday. Most of the foods they eat are locally and organically grown, vegetarian, and unprocessed. Their diet is essentially macrobiotic, as it is based primarily on whole cereal grains such as wheat, barley, buckwheat, corn, and brown rice, with fresh vegetables and greens, peas, nuts, beans, and fruits. Though they do eat some meat, dairy products, and poultry, these foods account for less than 1 percent of the diet.

We may not be able to adopt these peoples' level of activity (although many people feel we should), or their more rustic lifestyle, but we can adopt a more wholesome diet. In fact, nutritional research performed for the United States government has long recommended a more simple approach to diet. Two publications, *Dietary Goals for the United States* and *Diet, Nutrition and Cancer* came out in favor—in 1977 and 1982, respectively—of sweeping dietary changes, including more whole grains, whole-grain products, beans, fresh vegetables, and fruits, and less red meat, cheese, eggs, poultry, and highly refined foods that are lacking in fiber. The studies also recommend reducing salt, sugar, and fat consumption.

Medical and nutritional scientists believe such dietary changes can reduce the incidence of heart disease, hypertension, obesity, gallbladder and liver disorders, and cancer. The first report, issued by the McGovern Senate Select Committee on Nutrition and Human Needs, concluded that our present eating habits "may be as profoundly damaging to the nation's health as the widespread contagious diseases of the early part of the century."

Although these monumental studies received little, if any, attention from the news media at the time, thousands of people began turning to alternatives such as the macrobiotic diet to prevent illness and improve their health. Several well-known physicians, including Dr. Keith Block, a medical and nutritional consultant for CBS radio in Chicago, and Dr. Robert Mendelsohn, former medical director of the American International Hospital in Zion, Illinois, praised the macrobiotic diet as a ray of hope in the prevention of illness.

Drs. Edward Kass and Frank Sacks of Harvard University reported in the

American Journal of Epidemology, May 1974, that the macrobiotic diet normalized blood pressure. Their study of 210 individuals who switched to macrobiotics showed that the largely vegetarian diet was effective in bringing high blood pressure down to normal levels and that it maintained these levels far more effectively than the diet eaten by the average American.

A year later, *The New England Journal of Medicine* published another study by Drs. Kass and Sacks, this time stating that people who switched to the macrobiotic diet had healthier-than-average blood fat and cholesterol levels, despite having eaten the typical modern diet (which tends to elevate blood fat and cholesterol levels) most of their lives. In 1982, J. T. Knuiman and C. E. West confirmed Drs. Kass and Sacks's findings in their own research, which compared the total blood fat and cholesterol levels of macrobiotic, vegetarian, and nonvegetarian males. Their report was published in the journal *Atherosclerosis*.

The success of the macrobiotic diet in controlling blood pressure, fat, and cholesterol levels has made it medically credible. Some physicians are now recommending it to their patients along with standard medical treatments. In fact, at Boston's Lemuel Shattuck Hospital, wholesome macrobiotic meals are available to the staff and some patients. In Linho, Portugal, a group of prisoners have been given the opportunity to eat macrobiotically. Chico Varatojo, director of a macrobiotic center for the prison, feels that the poorly balanced nutrition of the conventional diet is largely responsible for crime and delinquency in modern society.

Unlike most other diets, macrobiotics has continued to grow and expand its sphere of influence for well over fifty years. Macrobiotic educators have been pioneers of the natural and organic foods revolution. Today, there are more than 500 learning centers teaching macrobiotics worldwide. In just about any large city, from Dublin to Dallas and from Athens to Atlanta, you will find people following the macrobiotic way. In many cities you will find one or more macrobiotic restaurants or restaurants that serve macrobiotic meals. Many individuals throughout the world have tried macrobiotics and discovered that it truly helped them to overcome poor health, even if they had been suffering for some time. They credit three factors as contributing to successful recovery:

1. The proper quality, quantity, and combination of well-prepared food;
2. Regular exercise; and
3. A positive mental outlook.

These aspects of the macrobiotic way are the focal points of this book. In the chapters that follow, you will learn what the macrobiotic diet consists of, how it compares to the diet currently eaten in many parts of the world, and exactly how you can use the macrobiotic diet and lifestyle to improve your health and that of your family.

ONE

The Way to Better Health

The macrobiotic approach to diet, exercise, and living can lead to better health for you and your family. If you choose to eat macrobiotically and follow the other suggestions in this book, you will reap the rewards of an active, intelligent, energizing approach to life. You will discover richness and harmony in nature, even amidst the pressures and hazards of our complicated world.

Macrobiotic philosophy teaches that a wholesome diet is the most direct path to good health, so the first part of this book is directed to examining the role of nutrition in the macrobiotic way. More so than any other approach to diet, macrobiotics appreciates and emphasizes individual differences such as where you live, what you do, and your present state of health.

Based on the philosophic principles of balance and harmony, the idea behind the diet is simple: your climate or geographical location, activity level, and physiology determine your nutritional needs. In making dietary choices, these factors are far better guides to follow than general nutritional and caloric tables.

In addition, macrobiotics points out the harmful effect modern methods of food processing and refining have upon our physical and mental health.

The macrobiotic diet uses only whole foods and foods that are processed by traditional methods.

WHOLE, UNPROCESSED FOODS

Unlike the people of Hunza, Vilcabamba, and other traditional cultures, who eat locally grown whole grains, fresh vegetables, and fruits, with few (if any) processed foods containing chemical additives, Americans have come to rely primarily on processed foods. As Dr. Alexander G. Schauss noted in his book *Diet, Crime, and Delinquency*, "The U.S. had the dubious distinction of becoming the first nation on earth to consume processed foods for more than 50 percent of its diet." Samuel Epstein, M.D., in *The Politics of Cancer*, tells us that the average American now consumes nine pounds of chemical additives per year, in the form of preservatives, artificial colorings and flavorings, and texture agents. This "American" diet is actually fairly typical of the average diet in other affluent industrialized nations as well. Yet, as the longevity and general good health of people whose diets contain few processed foods attest, the use of chemical food additives is not necessary for the maintenance of good health.

An excess of calories and saturated animal fats, combined with both the depletion of nutrients through food and the heavy use of food additives, is largely responsible for the staggering rate of health problems in many Western nations. The National Center for Health Statistics estimates that nearly one in every two Americans has a chronic condition that may result in disease of some sort. To reverse this situation, the macrobiotic diet recommends eating whole foods, primarily of plant origin, which are lower in calories, contain less saturated fat and no chemical additives, and require little or no processing.

LOCALLY GROWN FOODS

Each region of the United States (and of the world), through its geography and climate, places certain demands and stresses on the people who live there. Eating foods that are grown in the same conditions as those in which we live enables us to adapt more successfully to the changes taking place around us. A person living in a place with a cold, wet climate, such as Scotland or Ireland, would do well to eat the oil-rich oats that have traditionally been consumed in those places. Someone living in the southern United States, on the other hand, would be better off eating brown rice or the sweeter corn products grown in that region.

As much of our food as possible should be native to the area in which we live. For a New Englander to eat Florida oranges or Costa Rican bananas is to ignore the close connection between the body and its immediate environment, thus inviting seasonal imbalances such as colds and flu, and possibly more serious illness.

Most residents of the United States and Canada live in the temperate zone, north of the tropic of Cancer and south of the Arctic Circle. The foods that grow naturally in the temperate zone—especially whole grains, beans, seeds, vegetables, and some fruits—are balanced nutritionally for those of us who live where they are grown and harvested.

THE MACROBIOTIC DIET IN PERSPECTIVE

A three-way comparison of the macrobiotic diet with the one eaten in modernized societies and the one recommended by a government panel in the publication *Dietary Goals for the United States* is illustrated by Figure 1.1.

The macrobiotic diet is composed of whole foods. Most of the food energy comes from complex carbohydrates. On the macrobiotic diet, proper cooking methods preserve nutrients and enhance flavor in foods. Highly processed foods containing additives, commercial salt, and cane or beet sugar are avoided as much as possible. Dairy products, red meat, poultry, and foods containing these ingredients are generally not recommended for people living in temperate climates.

The *Dietary Goals* recommendations do not exclude heavily processed

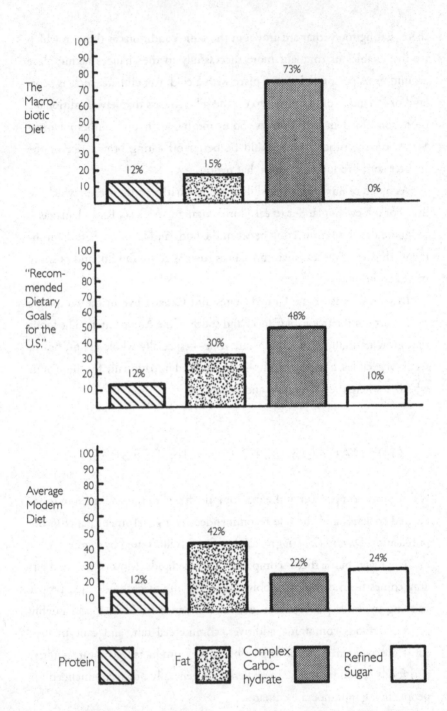

Figure 1.1 Three-Way Comparison of Macrobiotic and Other Diets

food items containing additives and preservatives. This diet is still too high in saturated fats, cholesterol, and highly refined vegetable fats to be considered optimally healthful. No special recommendations are made on cooking procedures or on balancing the diet. Yet these recommendations are a tremendous improvement over the way most of us eat now.

The modern diet relies heavily on processed and synthetic foods. It is much too high in saturated animal fats, cholesterol, and highly refined vegetable fats, and it is deficient in complex carbohydrates, fiber, and natural vitamins and minerals. Excessively high in salt, sugar, and chemical additives (some 3,500 have found their way into our food supply), the modern diet is increasingly subject to criticism from a standpoint of nutritional quantity and quality.

THE STANDARD MACROBIOTIC DIET

The macrobiotic diet consists of the following:

- 50 to 60 percent whole grains and whole-grain products;
- 20 to 30 percent locally grown (and, if possible, organically grown) vegetables;
- 5 to 10 percent beans and sea vegetables;
- 5 to 10 percent soups; and
- 5 percent condiments and supplementary foods, including beverages, fish, and desserts.

Figure 1.2 shows the proportions of the diet in graphic form.

Many of the foods that form an important part of the standard macrobiotic diet may be unfamiliar to you. These foods, and the menu shown below, will become more meaningful as you read this book and sample the recipes. On the macrobiotic diet, you can look forward to delicious and healthful eating as a way of life. If you would like to find out more about macrobiotic foods right away, turn to the Glossary on page 240.

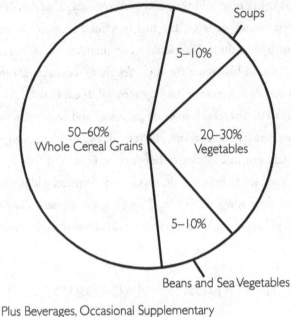

Figure 1.2   *General Proportions of the Macrobiotic Diet*

Although red meats, poultry, and dairy products, and dishes prepared with these foods, are generally not recommended for people in temperate climate zones, the macrobiotic diet need not be completely vegetarian. It includes small amounts of white-meat fish and certain shellfish. Richly nourishing tofu and tempeh (soy products that are minimally processed without chemicals, using traditional methods) are used in place of other animal foods. Seitan, a protein-rich wheat product; amasake, a sweet milklike drink made from brown rice; and a number of other supplementary foods that we will discuss more fully later on, are also included in the diet, often in place of meat and dairy products. Figure 1.3 outlines a sample of a day's macrobiotic menu.

In macrobiotics, whole foods are eaten as close to their natural form as possible. In place of refined grains or flours, we that suggest you use brown rice with only the outer hull removed, whole oats, whole rye, whole wheat, corn, buckwheat, and millet. Flours made from whole wheat, rye, buckwheat, and corn can replace white flour for making breads and pasta. Wholegrain breakfast cereals can be made from whole or rolled oats, freshly ground cornmeal, brown rice, and so on. A typical day's menu might look something like the one in Figure 1.3.

BREAKFAST

Oatmeal

Whole-wheat sourdough toast with apple butter

Bancha tea

LUNCH

Cucumber sushi and tempeh-sauerkraut sushi

Boiled salad with tofu dressing

Bancha tea with lemon

DINNER

Miso soup

Baked sole with rice

Grated daikon with toasted nori strips

Quickly boiled watercress and carrots with umeboshi-scallion dressing

Couscous cake with pear sauce

Grain coffee

SNACK (OPTIONAL)

Roasted seeds or nuts with raisins, rice balls or rice cakes, homemade popcorn, seasonal fruits (cooked, dried, or fresh), mochi cakes (made from sweet brown rice), or unleavened whole-wheat crackers

Figure 1.3   Sample Macrobiotic Menu for One Day

Denmark's "Macrobiotic Experiment"

During World War I, Denmark was blockaded, and widespread food shortages and malnutrition were a very real threat. Mikkel Hindhede, superintendent of the Danish State Institute of Food Research, was appointed food advisor to the Danish government. Hindhede not only solved the problem, but also achieved a complete reversal of the situation.

In the years before the war, Denmark imported inexpensive grain. Danish farmers bred pigs, cattle, and poultry, and sent eggs and butter to England. The Danes themselves were big eaters of meat and eggs. After the blockade, however, their grain supply was cut off, and there were more than 5 million grain-eating domestic animals and 3.5 million people to feed.

Immediately, Hindhede ordered that four-fifths of the pigs and one-fifth of the cattle be killed, so that more grain would be available for human consumption. In addition, consumption of pork and other meats was reduced or eliminated altogether. Hindhede also limited the production of alcoholic beverages, knowing that the grain used to make them could be better used to make a special whole-meal bread called *kleiebrot.* The Danes began to eat more porridge, fresh greens, vegetables, peas, beans, and fruits, and lesser amounts of milk and butter.

From October 1917 to October 1918, the most trying period of the war, Denmark became the healthiest nation in Europe. In one year on a diet similar to the macrobiotic diet, the cancer rate dropped by 60 percent and the death rate fell more than 40 percent. After the war, the Danes adopted their former diet and the mortality rate quickly returned to prewar levels.

The Best Foods You Can Eat

Do you avoid starches because you have heard that they are fattening? You may be surprised to learn that the complex, natural starches found in whole grains, such as brown rice and whole wheat, and in vegetables are in reality the best foods we can eat. Natural foods that contain complex carbohydrates are energy foods. Compared with proteins or fats, complex carbohydrates provide the body with more easily usable fuel for energy and leave behind fewer waste products.

Nearly everyone eats carbohydrates in some form at each meal. However, in our modern world, where processed and refined foods are readily available, up to half of the carbohydrates eaten by the average individual are supplied in the form of simple carbohydrates. The problem is that simple, refined carbohydrates can damage our health.

COMPLEX VERSUS SIMPLE
CARBOHYDRATES

A doughnut and coffee with cream and sugar in the morning or a candy bar in the afternoon may seem to give you a lift, but in reality these simple carbohydrate foods cause fatigue within a few minutes, when the sugar leaves the bloodstream. What happens is that the blood insulin level shoots up to counteract the overly quick release of sugar. This brings the blood sugar level down, way down, so that you start feeling tense and hungry for more sugar. Day after day, your body takes an uncomfortable roller-coaster ride, and your emotions can't help rising and falling along with it.

The macrobiotic diet replaces simple carbohydrates with more complex, slower-burning ones. Brown rice, for example, releases a continuous stream of glucose into the blood at a rate of about two calories per minute. The sugar in a candy bar is burned more quickly, releasing thirty or more calories per minute. Simple sugars such as honey, refined white sugar, and even fruit sugars are absorbed quickly because they are digested without the use of pancreatic enzymes, but they do not provide long-lasting energy. A macrobiotic meal of whole grains, vegetables, and beans will release its energy over a period of hours, without resulting in wide swings of mood or hunger for sweets.

ENERGY FOOD VERSUS BUILDING FOOD

Carbohydrates give us energy, whereas proteins help us to build and renew cells, muscles, and tissues. Even though the body contains a large amount of protein, our primary dietary need is for energy to maintain a balanced internal state. Carbohydrates must be supplied continuously in the diet because the body can store only small reserves of them. Only when the supply of carbohydrates is insufficient, as in starvation, does the body begin to break down proteins for energy.

The people of Hunza, well-known for their overall good health and longevity, get about 75 percent of their total caloric intake from complex carbohydrates, with the other 25 percent coming from proteins and fats. The ratio of complex carbohydrate to protein in their diet is about six or seven to one—identical to the macrobiotic diet. In contrast, the diet in many parts of the world contains about 12 percent protein and only 22 percent complex carbohydrates—about a two-to-one ratio, as you saw in Figure 1.1.

This means the average individual's body must work much harder, because it is forced to convert a portion of the fats and proteins consumed into energy. In addition, these conversions create waste products that must be acted upon by the liver and kidneys and eliminated from the body. The mainstays of the macrobiotic diet, on the other hand, are clean-burning complex carbohydrates that are converted by the body into glucose for energy, carbon dioxide that is exhaled, and water.

SWEET LOW, SWEET HIGH

The quality of the carbohydrates consumed is just as important as the quantity. A lack of complex carbohydrates, along with an excess of simple carbohydrates, is largely responsible for the problem of hypoglycemia (low blood sugar). Hypoglycemia first reveals itself as insatiable hunger, which may persist even on a full stomach. Fatigue, excessive perspiration, yawning, shaking, and emotional instability are a few of the other symptoms.

More than 10 million Americans suffer from hypoglycemia, some of them without ever knowing it. At first glance this would appear to be an absurdity: How could so many people have low blood sugar while consuming an average of nearly two pounds of sugar a week? If you recall our discussion of simple carbohydrates, you can see how it is the sugar itself that causes the problem.

Since sugar, in the form of glucose, supplies energy to the whole body, a lack of it can weaken every organ, including the brain, which depends on sugar to function properly. When too much sugar is eaten, however, it actually reduces the amount of sugar available to the body for energy.

The islets of Langerhans are tiny glands located in the pancreas that are responsible for the production of the hormone insulin. They become over-stimulated when there are excessive quantities of fast-burning sugar in the diet. For example, when a person with hypoglycemia consumes a candy bar or soft drink, the islets spurt insulin into the blood, lowering blood sugar levels and depleting stores of glycogen (a source of quick energy held in reserve in the liver). Unable to increase the blood sugar level without glycogen, the liver sends an SOS to the brain for help—and all of a sudden the hypoglycemic person craves more sugar. If additional sugar is consumed, the cycle is repeated. If not, the body secretes the hormone adrenaline, which, among other things, makes sugar available for energy in emergencies. The release of adrenaline is in part responsible for the symptoms mentioned earlier. And even though doctors may tell their patients with hypoglycemia not to eat sugar, many still do, because they do not understand why it is bad for them.

The standard recommendation for people with hypoglycemia is to follow a high-protein diet. In the short run, this seems to work fine. Every time such individuals feel a craving for sugar, they are instructed to eat a high-protein item to satisfy it. With a short supply of glycogen in the liver, the body is forced to convert protein into glucose for fuel. Making this conversion requires a tremendous amount of energy, and after a few weeks, a hypoglycemic person often finds it impossible to follow a high-protein regimen. Totally exhausted and craving sweets more than ever, he or she goes off the diet.

Years of experience in working with people who suffer from hypoglycemia has led me to a different approach to the problem. People with this condition need no more protein than anybody else. What they need most is the same thing we all need to have plenty of—fuel for energy, in the form of complex carbohydrates. It is best for those suffering from hypoglycemia to avoid sugar and refined foods. Moreover, hypoglycemic individuals may need to eat smaller, more frequent meals for a time. This is a relatively simple transition once you decide to do it, because the absolutely safe form of sugar, slowly released by the macrobiotic diet, replaces lost energy and reduces the craving for sweets. Every situation and every individual is different, however. Any questions regarding your personal needs should be brought to a trained macrobiotic counselor.

The Sweet Life of a Sugar Junkie

For years, my friend William Dufty, radio personality and author of *Lady Sings the Blues*, loved to eat sugar. "I must have been hooked very early," he says, "because my earliest memories of mealtime at home with the family was a kind of purgatory of meat and potatoes which I suffered through in order to get to heaven: a sweet dessert."

It wasn't until years later, though, while seated next to actress Gloria Swanson at a New York luncheon press conference, that Bill awoke to his problem. He was about to drop a sugar cube into his coffee when Gloria whispered, "That stuff is poison, I won't have it in my house, let alone my body." The conversation that followed stayed on his mind for days. He was overweight and felt lousy much of the time.

After Bill met Gloria and discovered macrobiotics, he gave up eating sugar and went on to write about his experiences. In the introduction to his book *Sugar Blues*, he writes:

> One night, in one sitting, I read a little book that said very simply if you're sick, it's your own fault. Pain is the final warning. You know better than anyone else how you've been abusing your body, so stop it. Sugar is poison, it said, more lethal than opium and more dangerous than atomic fallout. Shades of Gloria Swanson and the sugar cube. Hadn't she told me everyone has to find out themselves—the hard way? I had

nothing to lose but my pains. I began the next morning with firm resolve. I threw all the sugar out of my kitchen. Then I threw out everything that had sugar in it, cereals and canned fruit, soups and bread. Since I had never read any labels carefully I was shocked to find the shelves were soon empty; so was the refrigerator. I began eating nothing but whole grains and vegetables . . .

I had it very rough for about twenty-four hours, but the morning after was a revelation. I went to sleep with exhaustion, sweating and tremors. I woke up feeling reborn. Grains and vegetables tasted like a gift from the gods.

The next few days brought a succession of wonders. My rear stopped bleeding, so did my gums. My skin began to clear up and had a totally different texture when I washed. I discovered bones in my hands and feet that had been buried under bloat. I bounced out of bed at strange hours in the morning. My head seemed to be working again. I had no problems anymore. My shirts were too big. So were my shoes. One morning I discovered my jaw.

To make a long, happy story short, I dropped from 205 pounds to a neat 135 in five months and ended up with a new body, a new head, a new life.

The "little book" that changed Bill's life was *Macrobiotics,* by George Ohsawa.

THREE

Protein and the Macrobiotic Diet

Proteins are complex molecules found in almost all living things. Whereas carbohydrates are the best source of food energy, proteins are the best source of raw material for the vital processes of growth and repair.

Proteins are the building blocks of the human body. They are found abundantly in the muscles, tendons, blood, and organs. The hair, fingernails, and skin are all made of protein. Yet it is not protein itself that we need in our diet, but the components of proteins known as amino acids.

In the process of digestion, the body breaks down proteins into amino acids. The amino acids supplied by foods, along with those recycled internally, are reassembled by the liver, creating the proteins required by the body for the repair of cells and tissues, for growth, and to maintain metabolic processes. Of the twenty-two amino acids needed to maintain health, eight of them, known as the essential amino acids, can be obtained only from food. The body is able to manufacture the others from various substances.

This chapter considers protein and the macrobiotic diet from two perspectives: how the quality and quantity of protein in the diet affect health, particularly athletic performance; and how protein consumption relates to the problem of world hunger.

PROTEIN SOURCES IN THE MACROBIOTIC DIET

The macrobiotic diet supplies protein, including the eight essential amino acids, from the best available protein sources—whole grains, beans, vegetables, sea vegetables, seeds, nuts, white-meat fish, and fruit. Other protein sources, such as red meat, poultry, and milk, generally contain a high percentage of substances that can contribute to coronary disease and other health problems.

Many people today eat far too much protein, and since foods that are high in protein are often high in fat, these people may be eating too much fat (especially too much saturated animal fat) as well. Excessive protein in the diet can result in accumulations of urea, uric acid, fat, and cholesterol in body tissues and in the blood. Excess acid and fat in the blood tend to wash away stores of essential minerals, such as iron, magnesium, zinc, phosphorus, and calcium, causing the bones and teeth to weaken. In addition, as the National Academy of Sciences publication *Diet, Nutrition, and Cancer,* suggests, high protein intake may increase the risk of cancer of the breast, colon, rectum, pancreas, prostate gland, and kidneys.

Table 3.1 summarizes the nutritional composition of various foods. The percentages for protein, fat, and carbohydrate are based on the total caloric value of the particular food. For example, in brown rice, 7 percent of the calories come from protein, 4 percent come from fat, and 89 percent come from carbohydrate. In the root vegetable daikon, 16 percent of the calories come from protein, 5 percent come from fat, and 80 percent come from carbohydrate.

On the average, about 12 percent of the total caloric intake on the macrobiotic diet comes from protein, 15 percent comes from fat, and 73 percent comes from complex carbohydrates. The way to achieve this ideal balance is to eat a variety of foods that offer an optimal amount of high-quality protein, without excessive amounts of saturated fats or cholesterol.

IF YOU'RE AN ATHLETE

The myths surrounding nutrition are at present only beginning to fade. Let us examine a few of them. It is commonly believed that in order to build up big, strong muscles you need lots of protein. This is simply not the case. Even a bodybuilder's need for protein is the same as anyone else's. It is prolonged, strenuous exercise, not protein, that builds and strengthens muscles.

Another common myth is that when you use your muscles vigorously in sports or exercise it causes them to deteriorate, so that extra protein is needed to rebuild them. But, as early as 1866, pioneering scientists clearly proved that strenuous activity involves no increased use of protein. Unfortunately, the prevailing nutritional viewpoint is that athletes need high-fat, high-protein foods for strength and endurance.

A practice known as *carbohydrate loading,* or carbo loading, is popular as a way of increasing stamina among long-distance runners and other endurance athletes. Carbo loading originated in 1967 when Dr. Per-Olof Astrand, an exercise physiologist from Stockholm, tested nine Swedish athletes for endurance on a stationary bicycle. After three days on a diet high in grains and vegetables, the athletes were, on average, able to pedal three times longer than they did after three days on a diet high in meat and animal fats. In measuring the level of glycogen (fuel held in reserve) in the athletes' thigh muscles, Astrand found 3.51 grams per 100 grams of muscle after the vegetarian diet, compared with 1.75 grams after the three days on the high-fat, high-protein diet. From Dr. Astrand's experiment, and others like it, the concept of carbohydrate loading emerged.

Carbo loading takes a week to complete. Seven days before an athletic event, the athlete trains until totally exhausted to deplete muscle and liver

Table 3.1 Percentages of Protein, Fat, and Carbohydrate in Food

FOOD	% PROTEIN	% FAT (UNSATURATED)	% CARBOHYDRATE
Whole Grains and Whole-Grain Products			
Barley, pearled	8	2	89
Brown rice	7	4	89
Buckwheat, whole grain	12	6	82
Buckwheat noodles	12	6	82
Cornmeal, whole-ground	7	9	84
Millet, whole	3	8	70
Oatmeal	13	16	72
Popcorn	9	11	80
Rye	11	4	85
Wheat, bulghur	10	3	82
Wheat, whole	5	13	81
Whole-wheat noodles	9	3	84
Vegetables			
Bean sprouts	27	5	68
Beans, green	16	8	76
Broccoli	27	8	66
Brussels sprouts	28	9	63
Cabbage	13	7	80
Carrots	7	4	89
Cauliflower	24	6	69
Celery	13	5	82
Collard greens	23	17	60
Corn, sweet	9	9	81
Daikon	16	5	80
Kale	28	21	51
Lettuce, romaine	18	14	69
Mushrooms	25	9	55
Mustard greens	23	14	62
Onions	11	2	88
Parsley	20	11	69
Parsnips	6	6	87
Peas, green	26	5	69
Pumpkin	7	7	85
Squash, winter	7	5	88
Rutabaga	7	2	90

FOOD	% PROTEIN	% FAT (UNSATURATED)	% CARBOHYDRATE
Vegetables			
Turnips	10	7	83
Watercress	29	13	57
Legumes			
Adzuki beans	23	3	74
Black beans	23	4	74
Brown beans	23	4	74
Chickpeas	20	11	69
Lentils	26	trace	74
Lima beans	20	4	75
Pinto beans	23	3	74
Soybeans	29	37	34
Split peas	24	2	74

Source: Based on data from the United States Department of Agriculture Handbook No. 8, *Composition of Foods*, and from the Japan Nutritionist Association.
Note: One value is given for both cooked and raw foods, as the percentage of protein, fat, and carbohydrate is not significantly altered by cooking. As the calculated values have been rounded to whole numbers and are affected by various other factors, the percentages given here may not total 100 in every case.

glycogen. For the next three days, he or she eats as many high-protein or high-fat foods (such as red meat, eggs, poultry, and milk) as possible, with a minimum of carbohydrates. For the three days immediately preceding competition, the athlete's diet consists of high-carbohydrate, low-fat, low-protein foods such as pasta, bread, grains, sweets, and so on, in small meals throughout the day. During this carbo-loading phase, the muscles and liver store a relative overload of glycogen, which is needed for stamina and endurance on the day of competition.

Though the practice of carbo loading has met with some success, it is not without its dangers. The high-protein, high-fat phase of the diet leads to the production of substances called ketones. These are toxic and can lead to dehydration and kidney damage. In addition, the carbo-loading phase may bring large amounts of fat into the blood. Should the athlete have an existing heart condition, the rise in blood fats could lead to a heart attack.

A DIET FOR ENDURANCE

The best way to improve athletic performance, especially endurance, is to adopt the macrobiotic diet. Since it is naturally high in complex carbohydrates, the muscles will store the optimal amount of glycogen, without shocking the system.

Herbivorous animals such as horses, giraffes, and antelope have greater endurance than carnivores such as the members of the cat family, who are known for their long, lazy naps. This relationship of diet to endurance appears to hold true for humans as well.

The Tarahumara Indians, who live in the Sierra Madre mountains of northwestern Mexico, are an example of almost completely vegetarian superathletes. Their diet consists almost entirely of beans, corn, squash, pumpkins, root vegetables, wild plants, and fruits, with only occasional animal food (about one percent of their diet). Yet they may be the world's greatest endurance athletes.

Their bodies are strong and lean, and they are great runners. In their local sport, a kind of soccer game played with an oak ball the size of a baseball, the players run a total of up to two hundred miles before the game ends. During the night, other runners light the path with torches. The runners stop only every dozen miles or so for food and water. William E. Connor, who studied the Tarahumaras extensively, found them to be remarkably healthy. He reported his findings in the *American Journal of Clinical Nutrition*.

Closer to home, a number of successful athletes and superathletes follow the Pritikin diet, which is high in complex carbohydrates and low in fat and protein, similar to the macrobiotic diet. A few of the athletes mentioned in

A Vegetarian Baseball Team

A Japanese baseball team climbed from the cellar to first place by switching to a macrobiotic diet.

When he took over as manager of the Seibu Lions, Tatsuro Hirooka prescribed a dietary change for his players, who had finished in last place the previous season. Hirooka limited their meat intake and banned polished rice and sugar altogether. Instead, he said, his players would eat unpolished rice, tofu, fish, and soybean milk. The following spring, he ordered them onto a vegetable and soy diet.

Hirooka told his men that meats and other "animal foods" increase an athlete's susceptibility to injuries. Natural foods, on the other hand, protect the body from sprains and dislocations and keep the mind clear.

The Lions took a lot of ribbing during the season that year. The manager of the Nippon-Ham Fighters—a team sponsored by a major meat company—called the Lions "the goat team" and sneered, "They are only eating weeds." But the Lions edged out the Ham Fighters for the Pacific League championship in what sportswriters called the "Vegetable versus Meat War," then went on to beat the Chunichi Dragons in the Japan Series. Seibu again won the Pacific League championship and the Japan Series the following year. Food for thought, isn't it?

Nathan Pritikin's book *The Pritikin Promise* (Simon & Schuster, 1983) are world-class marathon runner Rob de Castella, winner of the 1982 Commonwealth Games in Brisbane, Australia, and, the 1983 Fukuoka marathon in Japan; Martina Navratilova, the world's top-seeded women's tennis player for many years; David Scott, the greatest triathlete in the world (competing in a ten-hour swimming, bicycling, and running competition); Scott Molina and Scott Tinley, two of Scott's closest competitors in the triathlon; and Jack Stevens, former world-record holder for the 400, 800, and 1,600 meter races in the sixty-five to sixty-nine age group. Sports enthusiasts can undoubtedly think of many others.

PROTEIN SOURCES
AND WORLD HUNGER

Beyond the question of individual dietary needs, there is the larger problem of food shortage and world hunger. The heavy drain on the world's energy and natural resources points to the need for a wide-scale reevaluation of our attitudes toward, and dependence upon, animal proteins as dietary staples. In modern practice, whole foods are often concentrated into refined and relatively less nutritious products. An average fast-food meal is an example. It takes nearly ten pounds of grain to produce the beef from which a hamburger is made; thirty ears of corn to get the oil for French fries; four pounds of soybeans and a half-quart of milk to make a shake; more than one pound of beets to produce enough sugar to sweeten a dessert; a host of additives to improve the flavor, texture, and shelf life of fast foods; and two grams of salt to flavor them. In addition, many refined foods that are high in saturated fats and calories are low in naturally occurring vitamins and minerals.

In the United States, nearly 2,000 pounds of grain are consumed per person every year (directly and through food for livestock). People in the rest of the world average about four hundred pounds of grain per year. Dr. Jean Mayer, president of Tufts University from 1976 to 1992, was outspoken when it came to our dependence on meat as food. Dr. Mayer estimated that reducing meat consumption by just 10 percent annually would release enough grain to feed 60 million people.

Frances Moore Lappé, the author of *Diet for a Small Planet* (Ballantine, 1992) and coauthor with her daughter Anna Lappé of *Hope's Edge: The Next Diet for a Small Planet* (Tarcher, 2002), points out that North Americans, who make up about 7 percent of the world's population, consume more than 30 percent of the world's animal foods. She contends that producing meat to supply humans with protein is grossly inefficient, and shows how vast acreage of land presently used to raise livestock could feed up to twenty times more people if planted with food crops instead.

FOUR

Fats and the
Macrobiotic Diet

The human body stores any extra energy that is supplied by the diet as fat. Because the modern diet is too high in both fat and total calories, it tends to foster excessive weight gain. Sixty-four percent of adults—very nearly two out of every three—in the United States are overweight, and one-third of those qualify as obese. More than 50 million people in this country are either on a diet or are contemplating going on one. This chapter will compare the sources of fats in the modern diet with those in the macrobiotic diet. Several areas in which dietary-fat consumption is of particular interest—overweight, heart disease, and infant nutrition—will be discussed.

For many people, the struggle to maintain normal weight begins slowly. Between the ages of twenty-five and forty they accumulate an extra fourteen pounds or so of fat. In many cases, this gain of one pound per year occurs if only 40 extra calories (above the average of 2,000) are consumed each day. You can visualize the extra calories as just two level teaspoons of sugar per day. Twenty minutes of slow walking or ten minutes of brisk walking every day would help to neutralize these extra calories. A change of diet could eliminate them altogether. The macrobiotic diet includes more whole grains, vegetables, and beans than the typical modern diet does, and fewer sources of fat.

Most physicians agree that being overweight poses significant risks to health. Not because of any psychological drain it may have on the overweight individual, but strictly because being too heavy is a menace to physical health. According to the panel of scientists who reported to the Senate Select Committee on Nutrition and Human Needs a number of years ago, obesity increases the risk of developing heart disease, hypertension (high blood pressure), gallbladder disease, and certain forms of cancer. It also aggravates arthritis, damages the liver, increases the risk of hernia, and causes difficulty in pregnancy and childbirth.

THE MACROBIOTIC DIET
AND WEIGHT LOSS

Although many complex explanations are frequently offered for why and how individuals become overweight in the first place, it is really quite simple: They eat too much of the wrong kinds of foods and they don't exercise enough. The modern diet supplies about 42 percent of calories in fat, a great deal of it in the form of saturated animal fat. By weight, fats contain more than twice the calories of protein or complex carbohydrates. Food processing has also condensed many of the foods commonly eaten. Since their bulk (natural food fiber) is removed, it is easier to fit more food—and calories—into the stomach in less time.

On the macrobiotic diet, up to 10 percent of an average meal is bulk, compared with about 2 percent or less in the diet eaten by most people today. The added bulk gives a satisfied feeling of being full, without adding calories to the diet. It also helps the body to more quickly and efficiently eliminate the food it does not use.

Unlike the foods that make up the popular high-protein weight-loss diets, which tend to drain energy and stimulate cravings for sweets, the complex carbohydrates in the macrobiotic diet reduce cravings for sweets and other fattening foods, and provide plenty of energy as well.

Losing weight and then maintaining the desired weight are not difficult on the macrobiotic diet. In general, people who shun foods high in saturated fats (such as red meats, dairy products, and poultry) and simple sugars are trim—and tend to stay that way. Depending on how much you weigh now and the extent to which you adhere to macrobiotic principles, your weight should normalize in a matter of days, weeks, or months. As in William Dufty's case, fifty or more pounds lost over a period of months is not uncommon.

On the macrobiotic diet, as long as you eat until you are satisfied, two or three times per day, you will meet your bodily nutritional needs. You can generally expect to lose about one to three pounds a week. Of course, if you also begin even a moderate exercise program, your results will be enhanced. (There is more about exercise in Chapter 14.) As an added bonus, your blood cholesterol and triglyceride levels and your blood pressure should normalize as well.

THE FATS WITHIN

The excessive dietary intake of cholesterol and fats creates significant health risks. As you probably know, high blood cholesterol levels, a substance akin to fats, has been implicated in coronary disease. In the past few years, many people have cut down on the amount of saturated animal fats they consume and reduced their cholesterol intake. However, the consumption of highly refined vegetable oils and hydrogenated vegetable fats (oils saturated with hydrogen), such as those in margarine and vegetable shortening, has increased. We now know that hydrogenated vegetable fats contain a type of fats known as trans-fatty acids, and these have much the same effect on the body as saturated animal fats do. And while polyunsaturated and monounsaturated vegetable fats are considered more healthful by some experts, the total fat content of the average American diet is still too high, regardless of its food sources. Even unrefined vegetable oils, if consumed in excess, can create blood that is too rich in fat and cholesterol. Most often the result is artery damage or atherosclerosis, a degenerative disease characterized by the development of plaques and fibrous tissue lining the artery walls and, in most cases, eventually blocking the arteries. Cardiovascular or coronary artery disease, as this condition is commonly referred to, is the number-one killer in America.

THE MACROBIOTIC SOLUTION TO HEART DISEASE

The macrobiotic lifestyle has long been known to be beneficial for the cardiovascular system. Separate studies by F. M. Sacks, B. Rosner, and E. H. Kass in 1974 and 1982; J. G. Bergin and P. T. Brown in 1982; *The East West Journal* in 1980; and J. T. Knuiman and C. E. West in 1982, published in major medical journals, have shown the macrobiotic diet to be effective in reducing elevated blood fat and cholesterol levels to healthy levels. The diet had a similar effect on high blood pressure, returning it to normal. In a 1981 study conducted by Dr. Sacks and colleagues, twenty-one healthy "macrobiotic eaters" were given beef for thirty days to determine the effect of meat and saturated animal fat on normal, healthy blood fat and cholesterol levels. In two weeks, the subjects' blood cholesterol levels rose from an average of 140 milligrams per deciliter (mg/dl) before the test to 166 mg/dl after. Blood pressure also increased significantly.

Shortly after the individuals returned to the macrobiotic diet, their cholesterol and blood pressure returned to their previous levels. Clearly, the macrobiotic diet is a promising solution to several important risk factors for heart disease.

Of course, some fat is necessary and even healthful. The naturally occurring oils found in whole foods and oils that are extracted from whole foods without further refining are the most healthful types. In moderate quantities, they help to protect the nerves from degeneration, provide necessary lubrication, and ensure the health of cell membranes. They also serve as emergency fuel reserves, keeping the body warmer in cold weather and being converted to energy when stores of glycogen are low. A little oil used in making bread or to sauté vegetables improves the food's flavor and digestibility as well.

Of the polyunsaturated fats, unrefined corn and sesame oils are the most stable oils for use in cooking and baking. They are followed by safflower, olive, and a number of other oils. (There is more about this in Chapter 8.) Stability is the capacity of an oil to retain its freshness on the store shelf or in your cupboard. The naturally occurring vitamin E found in unrefined oils contributes to their stability by serving as a preservative against rancidity.

About 10 to 15 percent of the calories in the macrobiotic diet come from fats. This reflects an ideal balance.

FATS IN DAIRY PRODUCTS

The quality of milk and dairy foods today is very different from that consumed by traditional peoples. Pasteurization, homogenization, and the addition of synthetic vitamin D chemically alter milk products. In addition, traditional peoples such as the Abkhasians, who use some dairy products, almost always ferment them. Cultured products such as yogurt and kefir are superior to other dairy products because they are more easily broken down in the digestive process. However, even cultured dairy products are not usually recommended for regular consumption on the macrobiotic diet, because they contain excessive amounts of saturated fats and cholesterol.

Research published in *Diet, Nutrition, and Cancer*, a National Academy of Sciences report, has linked the fats in dairy products to an increase in the presence of cysts and tumors of the breast, uterus, and ovaries in American women. Japanese women, who rarely consume dairy foods and eat fewer saturated fats than American women, have a lower incidence of these problems.

In addition, many people find that dairy foods cause the body to produce excess mucus, which often manifests itself as postnasal drip, symptoms of allergies, breathing difficulties, and blockage or irritation of the sinuses. Avoiding or minimizing the use of dairy foods has, in many cases, caused a reversal of these and other related problems.

Allergies to Grains

The fats and proteins in dairy products may be responsible for some food allergies. Through the years, I have counseled many people who, for one reason or another, were allergic to whole grains. In my opinion, people who have allergies or intolerances to either the gluten or other components of wheat, oats, corn, noodles, cereals, or flour products have probably been consuming too many dairy products as well as too much sugar since birth. How much is too much? Almost any amount, if you have an allergy to whole grains. Most of the time, this problem begins in infancy.

Babies that are fed cow's milk or formula miss out on their mother's colostrum, the milk secreted in the first few days after an infant's birth. Colostrum is needed to create strong immunity and healthy intestinal flora (bacteria) before the baby is ready to digest solid foods. Formula-fed babies are much more prone to disease in childhood and to food allergies later on—especially if they continue to consume excessive amounts of dairy foods and sugar.

Years of eating these foods cause a change in the cells of the stomach and intestines, including the villi (small tentaclelike structures that are responsible for assimilating food). The entire body may adapt to the larger protein molecules found in cow's milk and the excesses of calcium and other nutrients it supplies. At the same time, it may develop adverse reactions to normally wholesome foods. We call these reactions allergies.

If you are currently allergic to glutenous grains—especially wheat, oats, or corn—try using brown rice or millet, which are lower in gluten, as substitutes. Also, increase the amount of vegetables you eat, and eat more beans and bean products as well. Gradually reduce the amount of dairy products and sugary foods in the diet until you are able to avoid them completely. After a few weeks, try eating a small amount of the glutenous whole grains. In time, it may become possible for you to digest and assimilate whole grains without any adverse reactions.

The Best Sources of Dietary Calcium

Many people who were raised on cow's milk have come to depend upon it as a source of dietary calcium, a necessary nutrient. However, as you can see in Table 4.1, which lists various sources of calcium in the macrobiotic diet, many foods other than milk are rich sources of this vital mineral. And since these foods are all of vegetable origin, they offer higher-quality nutrition for adults—they contain less saturated fat and cholesterol.

Calcium regulates heartbeat, blood clotting, and overall mineral balance. It also builds healthy teeth and bones. Osteoporosis, a progressive weakening of the bones, frequently leads to fractures and death. Women past the age of menopause are particularly susceptible to this condition. A number of different explanations have been offered as to the cause of osteoporosis, and in the past, it has been common to blame it on an inadequate intake of calcium. While this may play a role, it is in fact most likely due to high protein intake together with the excessive consumption of simple sugars. This modern diet causes calcium and other minerals stored in the bones to be reabsorbed into the bloodstream. So, even if you consume adequate amounts of calcium, you can be losing it at the same time. By supplying an optimum amount of protein and a variety of calcium-rich foods, and eliminating refined sugars, the macrobiotic diet can help remedy this condition without side effects.

Table 4.1 Calcium Sources

CALCIUM SOURCE	SERVING SIZE	CALCIUM (MG) PER SERVING	CALCIUM (MG) PER 100 G
Leafy Green Vegetables			
Broccoli, steamed	1 cup	136	103
Mustard greens, steamed	1 cup	193	140
Turnip greens, steamed	1 cup	267	184
Kale, steamed	1 cup	282	185
Collards, steamed	1 cup	357	188
Seeds, Nuts, and Beans			
Sunflower seeds	2½ ounces	45	120
Pinto beans, dried	4 ounces	67	135
Chickpeas, dried	4 ounces	75	150
Tofu	3½ ounces	154	154
Almonds	2½ ounces	167	234
Dairy Products*			
Whole milk	1 cup	291	118
Cheddar cheese	1 ounce	204	750
Sea Vegetables			
Dulse	2 tablespoons	**	296
Agar-agar	2 tablespoons	**	567
Irish moss	2 tablespoons	**	885
Kelp	2 tablespoons	**	1093

*Not generally recommended for use on the macrobiotic diet.
**No data available.
Sources: United States Department of Agriculture and Japan Nutritionist Association

MACROBIOTIC NUTRITION FOR INFANTS

Milk has always served as a vital link between generations. Through the mother-infant breast-feeding relationship, the foundation is laid for the unfolding of intelligence and human consciousness. Even today, the long dependency of the newborn upon its mother tightens the bond between them and ensures that the child grows up strong and healthy.

Research has proved beyond any reasonable doubt that mother's milk is best for newborn babies. Formula-fed babies are more likely to develop digestive problems and diarrhea. They also have a lowered immunity to illness and infection, and less of a chance of surviving the first years of life alive and well.

Mother's milk is the best way to protect infants from viruses and microbes. It gives them a solid immunity against infection. According to Arthur Guyton, M.D., a noted medical physiologist and the author of the *Textbook of Medical Physiology* (W. B. Saunders, 2000), mother's milk contains specific antibodies that combat the growth of undesirable bacteria and viruses. Leonard J. Mata and Richard G. Wyatt, in an article entitled "The Uniqueness of Human Milk," which was published in the *American Journal of Clinical Nutrition,* said that mother's milk protects babies against the bacteria rickettsia (which can cause fever and typhus); polio, influenza virus, and salmonella, microbes that can cause intestinal infection; and staph, strep, and other infections.

In addition, a child's intelligence may be limited by the use of cow's milk. Studies reported in an article by W. B. Whitestone entitled "Biological Specificity of Milk," published by La Leche League, have shown that breast-fed children develop better reading and spelling skills than their counterparts who are fed cow's milk. It is not so difficult to understand why this could be so.

All creatures are born at different stages of biological development. For example, many species of fish can swim and eat immediately after they are born. Horses and cows are able to stand just hours after birth. Human babies can do little more than suck and are totally dependent on their mothers for a much longer time than most other animals.

Using brain development as a guide, we can compare the different animals and their nutritional needs in infancy. At birth, the human brain is about 23 percent developed, compared with 40 percent in the chimpanzee and gorilla at birth. A calf's brain is nearly 100 percent developed by the time the calf first sees the light of day. The various animals continue to show different rates of brain development after birth as well. Within the first year of life, the chimp's brain is three-quarters developed, but it takes three years for the human baby to reach the same developmental stage.

Not needing much brain food, but rather food for bone and muscle building, the calf may gain seventy-five pounds in the first six weeks. Cow's milk is three times richer in protein and contains four times more calcium than human milk. Human infants, on the other hand, grow less than a pound a week during the first six weeks. An infant's need for protein and calcium is much less than that of a baby calf. However, his or her requirement for carbohydrates, which nourish nerve and brain cells, is much greater than the calf's—and human mother's milk contains nearly twice as much carbohydrates as cow's milk.

While the practice of giving newborn babies cow's milk has been abandoned in recent years, some mothers still introduce cow's milk when their babies are a few months old. This may lead to long-term health problems, as cow's milk is too rich in protein, calcium, and other minerals for human babies. This is because it is designed to support the growth and development of a 300-pound calf.

Children fed cow's milk may become bigger in size more quickly, but their internal organs become somewhat lazy, loose, and enlarged. As it is composed of larger molecules than mother's milk, cow's milk tends to overnourish the body and undernourish the brain and nervous system. Breast-fed babies are generally brighter, more sensitive, and more alert than those fed cow's milk.

In most parts of the world, little milk is drunk by children over two years of age. Only by a lifetime of constant milk-drinking have some Europeans and Americans developed a seeming tolerance for dairy foods. Part of the reason that many people continue to use milk, butter, cheese, yogurt, and ice cream is habit, and part is emotional need. Just as babies are reluctant to give up breast-feeding and the taste and texture of milk, adults tend to develop an emotional attachment to its substitutes. The addiction goes beyond the emotions, however; as we have seen, the body is changed physically by years of dairy use.

Macrobiotic infant care suggests that the mother decrease the amount of breast-feeding when the child reaches about six months of age, while introducing soft foods such as creamy cooked brown rice cereal, millet, mashed noodles, oatmeal, soft cooked and mashed beans, vegetables, sea vegetables, and fruit. During the next year, the child is gradually weaned to soft foods. Harder foods can be introduced at around twenty to twenty-four months. Fruits and whole-grain cookies replace candies and sugared foods in the macrobiotic diet, and children can enjoy them with tea or amasake (a fermented drink made from sweet brown rice) instead of milk. Soymilk or nut/seed milk, beans and bean products, and whole-grain drinks such as amasake make good replacements for dairy products during the transition to a more macrobiotic diet.

FIVE

Fiber, Fermented Foods, and Digestion

The increased consumption of refined foods, sugar, and red meats has led to a drastic increase in problems of the lower digestive tract. The average American diet is extremely low in fiber and this deficiency has an adverse effect upon the beneficial microbes present in the colon (large intestine). To prevent problems with elimination and the lower digestive tract, including colon cancer, macrobiotics suggests the use of whole foods such as whole grains, beans, and vegetables, which are rich in fiber, and fermented foods such as miso, tempeh, tamari, umeboshi, sauerkraut, and pickles.

Speaking before a group of doctors, British doctor Dennis Burkitt, M.D., an authority on dietary fiber, explained our failing health in simple terms. Americans, he noted, have small stools and big hospitals. That is, due to a fiber-deficient diet, Americans suffer from a number of problems of the digestive tract ranging from tooth decay to constipation and colorectal cancer, which is the third leading cause of cancer deaths in the United States.

Fiber is perhaps the least understood portion of the food we eat. For years it was believed to be a useless non-nutrient that should be removed from foods to make them more digestible and palatable. In recent years, however, doctors and scientists have extensively studied the role of fiber in nutrition. Their conclusion is that, on the average, we cannot live very healthy or long lives without it.

FIBER AND FIBER DEFICIENCY

Fiber is the skeleton of the plant—the part that provides structural support. Every plant cell is surrounded by a fibrous wall. Fiber also forms part of the seeds, leaves, and stems. It is not a single substance but is composed of three different groups of substances: pentoses, which are complex carbohydrates; cellulose, which is also a complex carbohydrate; and lignin, a woody component.

Whereas fats, proteins, and non-fibrous carbohydrates are almost entirely absorbed in the small intestine, fiber moves through the colon, or large intestine, virtually unchanged. Because fiber is not digested in the usual sense, Westerners have been refining foods to remove it for more than 100 years.

In reality, fiber affects the function of the entire alimentary tract, exerting its greatest influence in the colon. Fiber adds bulk to the feces, facilitating their transit through the intestines. It also inhibits the formation of toxins and the growth of certain harmful bacteria in the colon. By diluting the concentration of toxins, fiber also prevents the colon wall from being harmed.

Asian people and those living in developing nations do not suffer from bowel disorders to the same extent that Americans do because their diet is less refined and includes more vegetables and fiber-rich foods. The incidence of colon cancer in the United States is 900 percent greater than in Nigeria and 1,300 percent greater than in Uganda, two African countries in which the diet is traditionally high in fiber. Yet after two generations of living in the United States, people of African ancestry contract colon cancer at the same rate as other Americans. Second-generation Japanese-Americans living in

Hawaii, having left their traditional high-fiber diet, also contract colon cancer at the same rate as the rest of the American public.

MACROBIOTICS AND FIBER

There is much evidence suggesting that switching to a high-fiber diet can prevent eliminative disorders such as constipation, hemorrhoids, diverticular disease, colitis, and bowel cancer. Fiber-rich foods such as whole grains may also prevent tooth decay, diabetes, obesity, heart disease, high blood cholesterol levels, varicose veins, and liver and gallbladder problems.

The macrobiotic diet, which is high in fiber, is the best way to promote a number of positive changes in the body. When you eat macrobiotically, your colon muscles are strengthened. In addition, the stools become larger, less dense, and easier to pass. Also, the intestinal flora ("friendly" bacteria in the intestine) becomes more healthy and more acidic, preventing gas and putrefaction. Dietary change is not only more effective than laxatives in correcting problems of the bowel, but is also the only really safe and long-lasting solution there is.

THE FIBER CONTENT OF FOODS

Fiber is more abundant on the outside surfaces of whole grains, seeds, beans, vegetables, and fruits, than on the inside. The bran of whole grains and the skins of beans, vegetables, and fruits contain large amounts of fiber. This is one important reason why the macrobiotic diet recommends using whole rather than polished grains and unpeeled fruits and vegetables whenever possible.

Many people, recognizing the importance of fiber, use bran, which is 44 percent fiber, as a dietary supplement. However, the regular consumption of added bran is not recommended as it may irritate the colon wall and interfere with the absorption of nutrients provided by other foods. Whole grains, beans, seeds, nuts, and unpeeled vegetables and fruits have an ideal balance of fiber and other nutrients. By eating plenty of high-fiber foods, you will get three or four times the fiber supplied by the average modern diet. Table 5.1 compares the fiber content of various foods. Animal products have been omitted since most of them contain little or no fiber.

Table 5.1 Fiber Content of Common Foods

FOOD	% FIBER
Bran	44.0
Almonds	15.0
Soybeans	14.3
Green peas	12.0
Whole wheat	9.6
Whole-meal bread	8.5
Peanuts	8.1
Pinto beans	7.0
Beans, other	7.0
Raisins	6.8
Brown rice	5.5
Lentils	3.8
Greens (average)	3.8
Carrots	3.1
Broccoli	3.0
Brussels sprouts	2.9
Apples	2.0
White flour	2.0
White potato	2.0
White rice	0.8
Grapefruit	0.6
Orange juice	0.5
Sugar	0.0

FERMENTED FOODS

Equally as important as keeping the muscles and walls of the colon in good shape with a steady supply of dietary fiber is keeping the flora inside it healthy. Though little is known about the 50 trillion microbes inside our intestines, what we do know could prevent much suffering and save some lives.

When we digest our food, it not only nourishes us, but also feeds the bacteria in the intestines. Eating whole grains, vegetables, and, especially fermented foods such as sauerkraut, pickles, umeboshi plums, miso, tamari, sourdough breads, amasake, and tempeh leads to the production of lactic acid in the colon. This acid gently tones the colon and corrects the balance between beneficial digestive bacteria and those potentially harmful but active bacteria that cannot develop so effectively in an acid medium.

The protective action of lactic-acid–producing foods was pointed out in a study of Japanese-Americans by J. S. Clarke that was published in the *Western Journal of Medicine.* Clarke found that Americans of Japanese descent still living on their traditional Japanese diet, including about two tablespoons of miso per day and other traditional fermented foods, had a significantly different and simpler (less diverse) population of microbes in their intestines as compared with average Americans.

W.E.C. Morre and L. V. Holderman, writing in *Cancer Research,* also reported a lower incidence of certain illnesses, especially bowel cancer, in populations where the bacterial flora is simpler than ours. The rural Africans and the rural Japanese are good examples of people with a more simple diet who have few eliminative problems. A simple grain-based diet of mostly unrefined foods, combined with the regular use of lactic-acid–producing fermented foods, and minimal consumption of meat and dairy products, is the key to their relative freedom from intestinal disorders, including colon cancer.

Light and salty-tasting miso soup, made with miso paste and vegetables, is a popular broth that can be eaten at least once a day on the macrobiotic

Dirk Benedict's Battle

William Dufty, author of *Sugar Blues* (Warner Books, 1993), which blames sugar for all kinds of health problems, introduced actor Dirk Benedict to macrobiotics. Benedict says it saved his life. Here's his story:

I used to eat like a horse. I'd have venison steak, eggs, and pancakes for breakfast, meat loaf for lunch, and a big steak, potatoes, salad, and apple pie or a piece of cake for dinner. I ate what Hemingway wrote about. In college I was a 200-pound linebacker, but I had very bad arthritis in my knees, hips, and hands, and headaches, hair loss, and skin problems. Then, while I was in Sweden doing a movie, I quit eating meat and chicken, and within ten days the pains in my knees stopped. The next year I began building my entire diet around grains, and two years later, I stopped eating dairy foods.

When I gave up meat, I was floundering. I was reading books on diet and Eastern philosophy and medicine, pursuing alternative ways of caring for yourself but for strictly physical reasons. Then Gloria and Bill [Dufty] introduced me to the Oriental philosophy behind an alternate way of eating—macrobiotics. Yin and yang. The balance of opposing yet complementary forces. They saved me years of searching.

Soon after this, I was told I had prostate trouble. I'd had pain and was passing blood. But I'd already changed my way of eating and I was thinking in much healthier terms. I was so pleased, having thick hair and no arthritis. My whole body had changed. I just didn't believe this could happen.

One doctor told me I had a tumor of the prostate, and then I went to another doctor in New York who said, "Yes. Definitely." He wanted to slap me right into the hospital. Bill Dufty had gone with me to the doctor. The way Bill figured it: "If they decide you have a problem, you're never going to get out of there. They'll lock you up and go to work." Bill was right. After the doctor gave me the bad news, some people came in with forms to fill out to check me into the hospital. I backed out of the office and down the hallway with doctors yelling after me. It was a scene right out of *General Hospital.*

Then I went to see Michio Kushi in Boston. I had first met him three years before. He confirmed that I had a prostate tumor and said it was very important for me "to have good behavior" for the next four months by sticking with the diet. No cheating. I was not scared because I had been studying macrobiotics, and I believed completely in the principles behind it. Actually, I was excited by the adventure of it. Growing up in Montana, I learned: If the tractor breaks down, fix it. So I always have had that in my nature. It was dangerous, but I wanted to figure it out on my own.

I didn't know what I was in store for. I didn't know how painful the journey was going to be, how difficult. I know people who've tried macrobiotic treatment for a while, and then just gone back to their cheesecakes. Everybody wants to be cured, but they want it to be easy, and they want it to be fast.

When I learned I had a tumor—I refused to be tested for malignancy—I weighed 180 pounds. When I came out of the mountains of New Hampshire six weeks later, I weighed 155. I went to stay in a friend's cabin because I didn't want any distractions, any temptations, anybody calling up to say, "Let's go have a bagel." Well, all hell broke loose. Some days I felt on top of the world, and other days I couldn't get out of bed. Sometimes I couldn't walk up the stairs, and sometimes I'd ride, run, and chop wood for twenty-four hours.

I wore a swimsuit all the time. There was no one around and no full-length mirrors—so I was shocked when I put on a pair of pants and they fell right off. I continued to lose weight, down to 135 pounds, at which point there were people who wanted to get me into a hospital. I looked like exactly what I was—someone who was seriously ill.

I never did go into a hospital. Instead, I packed up my duffel bag and became a vagabond, traveling to Montana, Maine, California, New York City, Wisconsin, hitch-hiking across the country once and driving across twice. I wrote short stories, a couple of screen treatments, and a proposal for a TV series. Food was a problem, though. The only thing I could find to eat in restaurants was oatmeal. I'd ask for one bowl, then another, and finally I'd ask for it in a salad bowl. The rest of the time, I relied on a little cast-iron pot, cooking grains and vegetables in the open field.

I shouldn't have traveled. I should have stayed in one place and taken care of myself. My body was starving to death. I was not eating anything my body was used to. Because of the cancer fear, I was not cheating. Before that, I would have a little cheese, a little fish, bread, salad, but now all that was gone. I was eating only grains, so my body was living off my fat, and then my body was eating my muscles. It was taking the protein out of my muscles; in effect, I was consuming myself. I used to dream about hamburgers and steaks pleading with me to eat them, like a Walt Disney nightmare.

At one point, I was driving from L.A. to the East Coast, and I swung up to Montana to see my family. I probably shouldn't have done that. I had never told them of my condition. It doesn't matter now, but I couldn't say it then. When my mother, who works in a hospital, saw how thin I was, she pleaded with me to see a doctor. I left her and my sister sobbing in the backyard and went down the road to New York.

I began to feel I was getting better when the weight started coming back after about a year on the diet. I went up to 148. I continued to stick with the diet, and gradually reached the point that I felt I was beginning to recover. Ultimately, I got a passing grade from my doctor after extensive blood tests. I didn't have the tumor anymore.

With macrobiotics, you begin to sense what you want. Most mornings now I have Japanese miso soup—which is made with soybean paste, chunks of tofu, seaweed, and scallions—and a big bowl of oatmeal. I take my own lunch to the studio—some kind of steamed vegetable. I also eat a lot of pasta and winter squashes. From the world of vegetables, there's almost nothing I don't eat. About 60 percent of my diet is grain, about 25 percent beans and another 15 percent side dishes like nuts, seeds, fruit, and fish. That's about as wide as I go.

The thing this diet does give you is stamina and endurance. What it does not give you is tremendous bulk strength. It wouldn't be too good for Mr. T. Some weightlifter friends of mine recently helped me move furniture. In the beginning they were stronger, but after two hours, I was still strong and they were pooped.

And my love life has changed. I appreciate a different kind of woman. I think the whole *Playboy* thing is the result of a meat-eating mentality. It's a gratification that is purely physical. It doesn't incorporate the emotional, the mental, the spiritual aspects of the female. But it doesn't have to be like that. My weight now has stabilized at 155 to 160 pounds. At five feet eleven inches, I weigh what I weighed as a teenager.

Macrobiotics is not to be taken lightly. It's not like going to see Richard Simmons twice a week and bouncing around and eating your salad. If you want to try macrobiotics, get some literature on the subject and read it. If it makes sense, incorporate it to some extent. Maybe three times a week, instead of having meat, eat brown rice. The whole point of macrobiotics is to get control of your life, and then deal with it yourself. Life belongs to those who are willing to accept the responsibility for having it.

diet. Tempeh, another fermented food commonly eaten on the macrobiotic diet, is made from soybeans. Pickled cucumbers, which you can easily make yourself at home, are another favorite, as is old-fashioned sauerkraut made with cabbage and sea salt. We will have more to say about the uses and preparation of these and other fermented foods later.

SIX

Is One a Day Too Much?

Among nutritional and scientific circles, there are two opposing sides to the question of whether vitamin and mineral supplements are necessary. There are those who say it is foolish to use supplements, that the average diet supplies all the micronutrients (vitamins, minerals, and trace elements) that we need. And there are those who tell us it's better to use supplements because we have nutritional deficiencies due to poor diet and environmental stresses.

The American public has the highest micronutrient intake in the world, due to the widespread use of vitamin and mineral supplements. A recent survey conducted by the Food and Drug Administration (FDA) indicated that more than 60 million Americans believe that vitamin supplements are absolutely necessary for good health. In addition, the study reported that 20 million Americans believe that vitamin deficiencies can lead to almost all diseases, including cancer.

One of the reasons that vitamin supplements are so popular is the massive advertising and promotion they receive, mostly sponsored by large pharmaceutical companies and supplement manufacturers. Another reason is that there is some truth to the advertisers' claims. The human body does need vitamins and cannot do without them.

Vitamins are essential nutrients, not for energy purposes but for their ability to regulate chemical reactions in the body. They help to make the energy present in food available for use. Without any vitamins, we would starve. Without enough of the right kinds, our ability to process and use the nutrients in our diet is reduced and a variety of deficiency symptoms, including malnutrition, may arise. Many people inadvertently destroy many of the vitamins in the food they consume. For example, washing with harsh soap strips away the vitamin C that is part of the acid mantle protecting the skin. Sugar and alcohol can neutralize vitamins B_1, B_6, and folic acid. Smoking interferes with the body's absorption of vitamin C. Excess protein or liquid in the diet can wash a variety of other vitamins out of the body, while antibiotics, laxatives, antacids, aspirin, many prescription drugs, and stress destroy even more.

Many of the vitamin supplements on the market are synthesized from coal tar and other petroleum derivatives. And while the synthetic substances may be chemically identical or closely related to the natural vitamins in food, they may have only a fraction of the biological activity. Synthetic vitamins may substitute for some, but not all, of the functions of their natural counterparts. Synthetics may also have additional effects beyond those of vitamins found in foods. In fact, vitamin manufacturers warn us that large doses of supplemental vitamins A, C, D, and E, and the B-complex vitamins, can harm the body. In addition, the use of smaller amounts of these synthetic vitamin supplements may lead to a gradual buildup of vitamin toxicity. If you do choose to use supplemental vitamins and minerals, try to obtain natural supplements (derived from food sources) rather than synthetic ones.

VITAMINS IN WHOLE FOODS

The macrobiotic diet supplies all the essential vitamins in quantities equal to or greater than the daily reference intakes, or DRIs, without supplements.

The key foods in the macrobiotic diet—whole grains, as well as fresh vegetables and leafy greens, seeds, beans, and fruits, are among the most vitamin-rich foods known.

Vitamin A, which aids normal growth and development, is supplied in abundance in the macrobiotic diet in the form of beta-carotene, or provitamin A. Provitamin A is nontoxic even in large doses and is easily converted into usable vitamin A by the liver. Yellow and orange vegetables and leafy greens are excellent sources of provitamin A.

The vitamin B complex vitamins is a group of vitamins that work together. The B complex vitamins help the body to digest and use the energy in carbohydrates, as well as foster resistance to infection. Among the best natural sources of the B-complex vitamins are whole grains, which make up 50 percent of the macrobiotic diet.

Vitamin B_{12}, which is needed by the body in minute amounts (a few thousandths of a milligram per day), helps to prevent nerve and cell degeneration, and aids in the formation of red blood cells. Since it is not found in plant tissue, it is sometimes perceived as lacking in the macrobiotic diet. However, it is often found in association with bacteria or mold on the skins of organically grown fruits and vegetables. In cultures where food is grown organically and processed minimally, and where no eggs, meat, or milk is consumed, vitamin B_{12} deficiency is rare. In addition, two important groups of supplementary macrobiotic foods—seafoods (such as sea vegetables, shellfish, and white-meat fish) and soyfoods (especially tempeh and miso)—do contain small but significant amounts of vitamin B_{12}.

Vitamin C has come to be regarded by many people as a panacea capable of curing the common cold, heart disease, cancer, and a number of other ailments. There is, however, no real evidence that taking high doses of supplemental vitamin C does any of these things. It does protect the nerves, glands, and connective tissues from oxidation and aids in the absorption of iron. The macrobiotic diet supplies three to five times the DRI for vitamin C, which is 50 milligrams per day. The best natural sources of vitamin C are fresh fruits, leafy greens, broccoli, and other vegetables.

Table 6.1 Essential Vitamins and What They Do

The following table is intended to help you select the foods in your diet wisely. It lists good food sources for the most important vitamins, outlines their functions in the body, and compares the current daily reference intakes (DRIs; formerly known as recommended daily allowances, or RDAs) with the amounts supplied by a typical day on the macrobiotic diet.

Vitamin	Sources	Function in the Body	DRI (adult)*	Estimated Macrobiotic Diet Value†
A (carotene)	Alfalfa sprouts Apricots Carrots Dandelion greens Leafy greens Orange and yellow vegetables Parsley Peaches Winter squash	Aids normal growth, reproduction, and development. Aids skin, teeth, mucous membranes, and eyesight. Maintains resistance to infection.	900 mcg (3,000 IU)	4,437 mcg (14,789 IU)
B₁ (thiamine)	Beans Leafy greens Nuts Seeds Vegetables Whole grains	Aids assimilation of starches and sugars; builds appetite and energy. Aids digestion, the heart, and the liver.	1.2 mg	3.07 mg
B₂ (riboflavin)	Almonds Kelp Leafy greens Mushrooms Soyfoods Vegetables Whole grains	Improves resistance to disease. Aids normal growth and development. Improves skin and eyesight.	1.3 mg	1.85 mg
B₃ (niacin)	Kelp Leafy greens Legumes Mushrooms Nuts Sesame seeds Sunflower seeds Whole grains	Aids mental health and nervous system. Helps maintain appetite and adrenal health.	16 mg	20–30 mg

Vitamin	Sources	Function in the Body	DRI (adult)*	Estimated Macrobiotic Diet Value†
B$_{12}$ (cobalamin)	Bean sprouts Dulse Kombu Soyfoods	Prevents nerve cell degeneration. Aids formation of red blood cells.	2.4 mcg	5 mcg
C (ascorbic acid)	Broccoli Brussels sprouts Cauliflower Collards Fruits Kale Parsley Sprouts Watercress	Aids growth and development. Maintains tissues, joints, ligaments, teeth, and gums. Promotes healing and resistance to infection.	90 mg	236 mg
D	Fish Exposure to sunlight	Promotes normal formation of strong bones and teeth.	15 mcg (600 IU)	10 mcg (400 IU)
E	Leafy greens Nuts Seeds Vegetable oils Whole grains	Aids reproduction, the heart, and the utilization of fatty acids.	15 mg (22.5 IU)	20–45 mg (30–67.5 IU)
K	alfalfa sprouts leafy greens sea vegetables vegetables whole grains	Aids blood coagulation. Decreases the risk of hemorrhage in pregnancy.	120 mcg	300–500 mcg

Sources: *DRIs: The figures used are adapted from the DRIs established for adults by the Food and Nutrition Board of the U.S. National Institute of Medicine, 2001.

†Estimated nutritional content of the macrobiotic diet (for one person, for one day) is based on *USDA Composition of Foods Handbook No. 8.*

Abbreviations used in the above table:

IU: international units (a measure of activity, not weight)

mg: milligrams (a measure of weight)

mcg: micrograms (a measure of weight equal to 1/1000 milligram)

Vitamin D is not really a vitamin, but more like a hormone, since it is synthesized in the body. It plays a role in the body's absorption of calcium, and it is important to the health of bones and teeth. This vitamin is not normally taken in in sufficient quantities from food alone—it is formed as a result of sunlight's action on certain cholesterol-like substances on the skin. (Because their bones are still growing, children in particular need regular exposure to sunlight.) Fifteen to thirty minutes of facial exposure per day is sufficient.

Vitamin E is believed to be an antioxidant—a substance that protects important molecules and structures in the cell from being damaged by free radicals. Even though vitamin E deficiency has never been observed in adult humans, supplemental vitamin E is second only to vitamin C in popularity. Advertisers claim that taking supplemental vitamin E increases sexual endurance, prevents heart attacks, and promotes longevity. Again, there is no evidence to support these claims. The DRI for vitamin E, 10 milligrams per day, can be satisfied by the consumption of one cup of leafy greens. Whole grains, unrefined vegetable oils, seeds, nuts, and vegetables also contain healthful amounts of natural vitamin E.

As you can see, a varied macrobiotic diet provides more than enough vitamins to maintain optimal health, without the danger of vitamin toxicity or buildup. For a summary of essential vitamins, good food, and what the vitamins do in the body, see Table 6.1.

MINERALS

Almost as many people take supplemental minerals as take vitamin pills each day. Minerals are added to white bread, cereals, canned foods, and baby foods. They can also be found among the vitamins in many supplements. But as is the case with most supplemental vitamins, the minerals added to foods or found in pills usually do not come from food sources at all, but rather from mines and quarries (via laboratories).

Minerals that occur naturally in food are always combined by nature with specific amino acids, and sometimes with vitamins, too. The body easily recognizes minerals in this form and knows how to use them efficiently. As food additives or dietary supplements, however, minerals tend to confuse the body more than they help it.

When the body does accept a mineral element, it must then balance it with its overall mineral needs. This is because the balance among various minerals is often more important than the absolute level of any individual mineral. Taking too much of a particular mineral can set up a chain reaction that unbalances all the other mineral levels. This doesn't mean that taking an iron pill for a few days will cause illness. It probably won't make any difference. But if iron or other supplemental minerals are used over a longer period of time, they may upset all of the major mineral balances that are important to health.

Taking iron supplements to treat anemia actually may make the problem worse. When an individual takes an iron pill, his or her sodium level goes up due to adrenal stimulation. The elevated sodium lowers the magnesium level. This also brings the calcium down, the potassium up, and the copper and zinc down—ultimately lowering iron even further.

In other words, no mineral works alone; they all work in harmony to balance one another. Extreme diets, supplemental minerals, and some pathological conditions can overwhelm the delicate mechanisms that maintain the minerals in proper proportion. Healthy people who eat a balanced wholefoods diet will be able to keep their minerals in the proper ratio to one another. In fact, no matter what your physical condition is, food is the safest and best place from which to get all your minerals.

THE ROLE OF MINERALS IN HEALTH

The balanced minerals found in whole foods are extremely important. They help keep energy levels high, nerves tranquil, and muscles, heart, hair, and blood healthy. They are also important in the formation of bones, teeth, and nails. Moreover, minerals play a role in almost all physiological functions.

Table 6.2 Essential Minerals and What They Do

Mineral	Sources	Function in the Body	DRI (adult)*	Estimated Macrobiotic Diet Value†
Calcium	Daikon radish Dandelion greens Dulse Kale Kelp Leafy greens Nuts Parsley Sea vegetables Sesame seeds Soy foods Watercress	Builds healthy bones and teeth. Helps blood to clot. Regulates heartbeat and mineral balance.	1,300 mg	1,350 mg
Chlorine	Celery Green cabbage Kale Lettuce Parsnips Radishes Sea vegetables Vegetables	Aids digestion and elimination. Sustains normal heart activity.	Trace	Trace
Iodine	Fish Leafy greens Sea vegetables Vegetables (organically grown)	Stimulates the thyroid gland, which regulates the rate of digestion. Important for growth and development.	150 mcg	150–300 mcg
Iron	Beans and legumes Fruits (dried and fresh) Kelp Leafy greens Nuts Sea vegetables Seeds Tekka Whole grains	Helps to form hemoglobin and myoglobin. Aids oxygen transport to cells and prevents anemia.	18 mg	39.3 mg

Mineral	Sources	Function in the Body	DRI (adult)*	Estimated Macrobiotic Diet Value†
Phosphorus	Beans and legumes Fruits Nuts Pumpkin and squash seeds Sea vegetables Sesame seeds Sunflower seeds Vegetables Whole grains	Builds and maintains bones, teeth, hair, and nervous tissue. Assists cells in absorbing fats and carbohydrates.	1,250 mg	1,539 mg
Potassium	Beans and legumes Cabbage Chestnuts Dulse Fruits (fresh and dried) Kelp Leafy greens Nuts Vegetables	Maintains mineral balance and weight. Tones muscles.	—	3,666 mg
Sodium	Cucumbers Horseradish Leafy greens Miso Root vegetables Sea vegetables Sesame seeds Tamari	Aids digestion, speeds elimination of carbon dioxide, and regulates body fluids and heart action.	500 mg	2,560 mg

Sources: *DRIs: The figures used are adapted from the DRIs established for adults by the Food and Nutrition Board of the U.S. National Institute of Medicine, 2001.

†Estimated nutritional content of the macrobiotic diet (for one person, for one day) is based on *USDA Composition of Foods Handbook No. 8.*

Abbreviations used in the above table:

IU: international units (a measure of activity, not weight)

mg: milligrams (a measure of weight)

mcg: micrograms (a measure of weight equal to 1/1000 milligram)

Note: A dash signifies that no DRI has been established.

For example, not only do they serve in maintaining immunity from disease, but also in regulating blood pH (the relative acidity or alkalinity of the blood). Just as seawater can neutralize toxins streaming into it from the land, minerals in our blood can neutralize excesses of acid or alkaline ash, the residue left behind from digesting and metabolizing foods.

Under normal circumstances, our blood should maintain a slight alkalinity, having a pH between 7.3 and 7.45 (on the pH scale, below 7.0 is acid and above 7.0 is alkaline). As a result of metabolism, acids are constantly being produced. These must be neutralized by the alkaline elements in the blood in order to prevent acidosis (an overly acidic body system), ketosis shock, gout, and other problems. The more acid produced internally and the more taken in from food, the lower the reserves of alkaline minerals like calcium will become. After years of a diet high in acid-forming foods, such as red meat, sugar, poultry, eggs, tropical fruits, fats, and oils, the body becomes overly acidic. More calcium begins to leave the body than stays inside it, causing bones to weaken and teeth to decay.

Testing food for acidity or alkalinity is performed by burning the food and analyzing the ash that remains. If a food has an alkaline ash, it is alkaline-forming; if it has an acid ash, it is acid-forming. The confusion surrounding the question of acid- and alkaline-forming foods regards the effect these foods have on the blood.

Some foods that test acidic in ash—for example, whole grains, which have a mildly acidic ash—can actually have a slightly alkaline-forming effect on the blood. Alkaline-ash foods such as tropical fruits, on the other hand, cause an acidic reaction. Sugar, which also has an alkaline ash, and some vegetables of tropical origin, including tomatoes, create acidity in the blood as well.

Unlike the diet typical of many people today, the macrobiotic diet has a total pH value that is slightly alkaline-forming in the bloodstream. The result is a higher energy level, immunity from colds and flu, prevention of stomach upset, and stronger and more healthy bones and teeth.

Table 6.2 indicates good food sources of the essential minerals and details the functions of each in the body. It also compares the DRIs with the amounts supplied by a typical day on the macrobiotic diet.

Of all the foods we recommend you eat regularly, sea vegetables are the richest source of minerals. Millions of people all over the world still eat sea vegetables direct from the sea, and benefit both from the minerals they contain and the flavor they add to other foods. Table 6.3 lists the mineral content of the various sea vegetables recommended for regular consumption on the macrobiotic diet. The role of sea vegetables in the diet will be discussed more fully in the next chapter.

In this age of specialization, where the accumulated knowledge resulting from intense research is so great, it is easy to lose sight of the wholeness of life. This is not to say that knowledge of nutritional science is a waste of time. An understanding of nutritional needs can help us to better choose the whole foods we need and recognize when we need them. At the same time, we must

Table 6.3 Mineral Content of Various Sea Vegetables

The figures in the table below represent the number of milligrams of each mineral per 100 grams (about 3½ ounces) of sea vegetable.

Sea Vegetable	Calcium	Phosphorus	Iron	Sodium	Potassium
Agar-agar	567	22	6.3	—	—
Arame	1,170	150	12.0	—	*
Dulse	296	267	—	2,085	8,060
Hijiki	1,400	56	29.0	—	*
Irish moss	885	157	8.9	2,892	2,844
Kelp	1,093	240	—	3,007	5,273
Kombu	800	150	—	2,500	*
Nori	260	510	12.0	600	*
Wakame	1,300	260	13.0	2,500	*

Sources: United States Department of Agriculture and Japan Nutritionist Association.
Note: A dash signifies a lack of reliable data for a mineral believed to be present in a measurable amount. An asterisk (*) signifies that information is not available.

Up from Hypoglycemia—A Case History
Diane Sacolick's Story

Before I became very ill, I had several chronic health problems that I had accepted as a part of my life. The only efforts I made to improve my situation were to see doctors and have prescriptions filled. I was constipated most of the time, usually had a yeast infection, and had between three and six colds a year. I used the laxative Metamucil for constipation, tube after tube of the fungicidal cream Monistat for yeast infections, and antibiotics for colds.

Every year my bladder infections would increase in number and discomfort. After I saw three different doctors and tried eight different drugs, a urologist told me my periurethral glands were also infected. His only suggestion was an operation, which he said would be extremely painful and probably wouldn't help much. I decided to pass on the operation and convinced my internist to give me Macrodantin (a brand name for nitrofurantoin, an antibiotic), which had worked for a friend who had similar problems. The Macrodantin stopped the infections and the acute pain, and I took it daily as preventive medicine.

I needed to take Motrin, an anti-inflammatory, every four hours during my period or else, by the time four and a half hours were up, I'd be in tears from the pain in my abdomen. Even with the medication, I was uncomfortable and severely depressed during my period and found it very difficult to get through the day.

I had gone to Washington, D.C., in August to attend Georgetown University Law School. My body endured lack of sleep and poor eating habits remarkably well until October. Then I started to have occasional dizzy spells. I'd become depressed without having the faintest idea why. I came down with a cold that wouldn't go away and was bedridden for two one-week periods, sleeping up to twenty hours some days. The dizzy spells began to come more and more frequently, now accompanied by difficulty in breathing, blurred vision, and tears. The only advice doctors or nurses gave me at this time was to "take it easy," and one gave me a prescription for antibiotics. My throat, sinuses, ears, and nose were all infected at one point.

By December, I was unable to read and study for exams, so I deferred them until January. I went home to Manhattan. My family doctor could not find anything wrong with me.

At this point, I was so depressed that I started contemplating suicide. Since there was nothing wrong with me physically, according to the doctor, I thought I must be going crazy. I considered checking into a mental hospital, but I continued searching for an answer.

While I was home, my mother had a party and I met a woman there who had been diagnosed as hypoglycemic. She had some of the same problems. This was it! I thought. I took a glucose tolerance test a few days later. My worst symptoms appeared in full force both during and after the test: dizziness, blurred vision, breathing difficulty, crying spells. The doctors concurred in their diagnosis of my condition as hypoglycemia.

In early January I started the diet standardly prescribed for hypoglycemia by physicians—high in protein, low in carbohydrate. My daily fare consisted of six to eight small meals that included one of the following foods: milk, cheese, nuts, fish, chicken, red meat, or eggs. I drowned my fish, chicken, and eggs in butter because I loved the taste of it, and because a high-fat diet was supposed to be good for hypoglycemia, according to several books I had read. The rest of my diet consisted of low-carbohydrate vegetables such as mushrooms and lettuce. I completely gave up my smoking habit and my large intake of coffee, alcohol, diet soda, sugar, flour, and fruit at this time. I notified Georgetown that I would not be returning.

My condition improved somewhat. The depression lifted a bit and dizzy spells came less frequently. Yet although I was very strict on this diet, I still experienced very severe hypoglycemic symptoms at times. My mind was so clouded that I would constantly forget what I was going to say or where I put something. Many days I would just buy food and prepare my meals; this alone would exhaust me for the whole day. My fingers always had at least two bandages on them, sometimes three or four, as I burned and cut myself many times while cooking. I became afraid to walk outside by myself, afraid that I would collapse in the street. I stayed home most of the time and "gave it time." I gained ten pounds.

By early March I decided something more had to be done. I began a series of visits to an allergist. At his instruction, I recorded everything I ate and when I ate it for a week; I also noted what my symptoms were and when I experienced them. I wrote down what every object in my apartment was made of, as well as the name of every cosmetic and cleaning item I used. I spent hundreds of dollars on various tests, hundreds more on subsequent appointments.

Over the course of five weeks, I was diagnosed as having other problems besides hypoglycemia, including an overgrowth of *Candida albicans* (yeast syndrome), an acute allergic state, inhalant and chemical sensitivities, immune deficiency, an allergy to milk and milk products, and insufficient pancreatic enzymes and hydrochloric (digestive) acid. I stopped consuming all milk products. With every meal, I took digestive aids such as hydrochloric acid and KAL-N-Zyme (a food-based enzyme product). I bought nystatin, an antifungal, to combat the yeast problem, and purchased ten bottles of vitamins to boot. I felt much better, but still had very low energy and suffered occasional "attacks" of dizziness accompanied by breathing and vision difficulty.

I was not very comfortable with my new regime, and the next step was expensive allergy testing and rotating foods, which involves eating no one food more than once every four days. I knew this wasn't going to help me and couldn't bear the thought of doing it. When the allergist's assistant suggested that I remove all the plants from my apartment—as mold on them was suspected of causing my symptoms—I knew there had to be a better solution. My diet became more and more restricted and boring as I tried to figure out what was making me sick.

About this time, the Hypoglycemia Association, Inc. (HAI), of Maryland sent me a bulletin that included a description of the next meeting. Bill and Barbara Taylor were going to speak to HAI about macrobiotics. It appealed to me instantly. I was so sick of red meat and chicken. I read Dr. Anthony Sattilaro's book *Recalled by Life,* and I became very excited because I strongly sensed macrobiotics was going to help me.

After hearing the Taylors speak, I was more than ready to begin exploring macrobiotics. I made an appointment with Michael Rossoff, a macrobiotic counselor and acupuncturist in Bethesda, Maryland. After the interview and assessment, he suggested a dietary plan for my condition. The recommendations were for food, acupressure points, and books—not drugs or vitamins.

After three days of following these recommendations, my six months of dizzy spells and accompanying symptoms disappeared, never to return. I was elated. Within seven months of following the macrobiotic diet, most of my other problems also disappeared. I have no allergic reactions, I no longer suffer from constipation, and this is the longest I have gone in years without a cold, yeast infection, or bladder infection. That September, I had my first period without cramps in six years. This improvement was accelerated by a series of ten acupuncture treatments I received while maintaining my new way of eating.

I have never before eaten such a varied and fun "diet." Both cooking and eating are a great pleasure for me now. Instead of eating every two to three hours, I enjoy three meals a day. I'm no longer a slave to the clock. If I choose to, I can now wake up in the morning, exercise, and wait as much as three hours before eating, instead of staggering from my bed to the kitchen. I've also lost the weight I gained earlier this year.

My thinking is clearer, and I am happier, calmer, and more patient than ever before. At times I do get tense and impatient, and I still occasionally have trouble with fatigue, but—all in all—my health is improving much more quickly than I would have ever thought possible.

Another wonderful aspect of macrobiotics is the cost as compared with most alternative approaches to better health. Most of the food is inexpensive, especially when compared with meat and cheese. While I was on the high-protein diet I felt so deprived and unhappy that I would often "treat" myself to expensive cheeses and meat. Now there are no tests to take and no drugs or vitamins to buy.

And, of course, the value of increased energy and happiness experienced through macrobiotics is priceless.

consciously look beyond fragments of truth to view the wholeness of life. Individuals born into a traditional way of life see no such separation. Their food selection is merely a part of their whole history, culture, and dietary tradition. And with their whole diet, these people preserve the wholeness of their health. In keeping with these traditions, the macrobiotic approach brings wholeness to our diet and, therefore, to our health and our lives.

SEVEN

Key Macrobiotic Foods

The macrobiotic diet is in accord with the latest scientific evidence on diet and nutrition, yet the rich blend of tradition and common sense that lies at its core is perhaps an even better reason to eat macrobiotically. Since the advent of agriculture, about 12,000 years ago, the majority of humans have eaten a diet consisting of whole grains, whole-grain products, vegetables, and beans, with limited quantities of animal foods.

Following the agricultural revolution of the 1800s, the modern diet began to change rapidly. The abundance of inexpensive grain made animal husbandry profitable, and meat and dairy foods became widely available. The invention of the roller mill changed the way bread was made, by refining whole grains—separating the bran and germ portions from the endosperm. The prosperity of the early 1900s provided the average individual with access to refined foods and meats that previously were available only to the wealthy. During the past seventy-five years or so, our food supply has become increasingly artificial, and animal foods have gained in popularity. Macrobiotics favors a more traditional way of eating that emphasizes natural, wholesome foods.

In this chapter and the next, we will discuss the nutritional value, interesting aspects, and uses of macrobiotic foods beginning with whole grains.

WHOLE GRAINS: OUR SOURCE OF ENERGY

Human physiology has not adjusted well to the new habits of eating "fast foods." There is no better illustration of this fact than the growing interest in whole foods, especially whole grains. Thousands of years ago our ancestors began eating the nutritious fruit and seed combination we call whole grain. Since then, many cultures have adopted grains as their staple food. The ancient Chinese depended upon millet, buckwheat, and rice as their staples; the Aztecs and Mayans subsisted mainly on corn; the Egyptians grew some of the world's finest wheat; the early Europeans relied on wheat, rye, barley, and oats; the Britons relied on oats and wheat; the Hindus relied on rice and wheat; and a number of African peoples cultivated millet. Some of our ancestors even worshipped grain as a god of life, the fabric of which humans were made. The Japanese word for "peace and harmony" also denotes the eating of grains.

Whole grains are grains that are eaten intact. In whole grains, none of the edible portions (the bran, germ, and endosperm) are removed. On the macrobiotic diet, whole barley, buckwheat, brown rice, millet, oats, rye, and wheat are pressure-cooked, boiled, or baked into casseroles. Whole-grain products, ranging from sourdough whole-wheat bread to spaghetti are also eaten. Almost any refined grain product that you can find can also be made from whole grains.

Whole grains are composed of complex carbohydrates, proteins, fats, vitamins, and minerals in ideal proportions for the needs of the human body. The ratio of complex carbohydrates to protein in the macrobiotic diet is about seven to one. Whole grain itself also reflects this ideal balance, providing about seven times more complex carbohydrates than protein. Whole grains are also an excellent source of fiber, B-complex vitamins, vitamin E, and phosphorus, a key mineral and brain food.

Beyond their healthfulness, there is at least one other reason to use plenty of whole grains. Of all foods, they are probably the least expensive, because they are so widely cultivated. They cost less to grow—and to eat, per food value dollar—than red meat, eggs, dairy products, poultry, or fish. The

Table 7.1 Whole Grains and Grain Products

FOR REGULAR USE	FOR OCCASIONAL USE	TO BE AVOIDED
Whole barley	Buckwheat noodles (soba)	Baked goods containing dairy
Whole millet	Rice cakes	products
Whole wheat	Udon (whole-wheat	Refined grain cereals
Whole buckwheat	noodles)	Yeasted breads, crackers,
Whole rye	Corn grits or cornmeal	cakes, cookies, and so on
Other whole-cereal grains	Rice kayu (porridge) bread	White-flour products
Whole corn	Unyeasted whole-wheat or	
Whole short-grain brown	rye bread	
rice	Couscous	
Whole medium-grain brown	Rye flakes	
rice	Wheat gluten (seitan)	
Whole oats	Cracked wheat (bulghur)	
	Somen (sifted whole-wheat	
	noodles)	
	Whole-wheat crackers or	
	matzo	
	Long-grain brown rice	
	Sourdough whole-wheat or	
	rye bread	
	Whole-wheat pasta	
	Pounded sweet rice cakes	
	(mochi)	
	Steel-cut or rolled oats	
	Puffed wheat gluten (fu)	
	Sweet brown rice	
	Ramen noodles (whole	
	wheat, rice, buckwheat)	
	Tortillas	

grains most recommended for regular use are barley, brown rice, buckwheat, corn, millet, oats, and wheat. Table 7.1 provides a more complete list of whole grains and grain products.

VEGETABLES

The word *vegetable* is derived from a Latin word meaning "able to live (or grow)," "vigorous," "lively," and "full of life." In keeping with their namesake, vegetables (including sea vegetables) supply the full spectrum of vitamins and minerals we need to live and grow in good health.

Vegetables provide the macrobiotic diet with a variety of colors, tastes, and textures. Cut into different shapes and cooked in a variety of ways, vegetables add freshness and lightness to dishes containing whole grains and beans. In smaller amounts, pickled or raw vegetables are also used.

Homegrown vegetables are best. They are fresh, full of flavor, and free from synthetic fertilizers or sprays. In season, they can be prepared in countless ways, both cooked and raw. At the harvest, when homegrown and local produce is abundant and inexpensive, fresh vegetables can be dried, pickled, or stored in a cold cellar for use through the winter.

In the winter, summer vegetables such as cucumbers and string beans are often shipped from warm areas like Mexico or Florida to colder climates. But these vegetables have lost the flavor natural to the colder environment; they are out of season and out of balance with local physiological needs. If you live in a colder climate, it is better to buy vegetables such as winter squash, cabbage, and root vegetables, which are more suited to cooler weather, or to store local vegetables for use during the winter months.

There are more than 100 edible vegetables, many of which are included in the three main groups of vegetables recommended on the macrobiotic diet—green leafy vegetables, root vegetables, and ground vegetables.

Green Leafy Vegetables

Fresh leafy greens like collards or kale are among the most nutritious foods available. Pound for pound, they provide more vitamins, minerals, and proteins than meat does—for a fraction of the cost. If you are not in the habit of eating fresh greens, you can begin by adding them to soups or sautéed vegetables, until you can also enjoy them cooked separately, served with whole grains and beans.

Greens are important to the macrobiotic diet for several reasons. One reason is that they are rich in chlorophyll—a protein compound that aids in creating healthy red blood cells. Leafy greens are also an excellent source of vitamin C, calcium, and alkaline minerals. These neutralize excess acidity in the blood. One reason it is recommended that fish be eaten along with greens and a little grated raw daikon (white radish) is that the latter two provide vitamins and minerals that help us to digest and use the nutrients in the fish better. Fresh greens enjoy a long growing season and are available locally in many parts of the country year-round.

Root Vegetables

As a group, the root vegetables are good sources of vitamins and minerals, and excellent suppliers of complex carbohydrates. Dense and compact root vegetables, such as carrots, rutabagas, and parsnips, are rich in minerals and complex carbohydrates, and, compared to the leafy vegetables, require greater digestive effort. In the process, they promote warmth and improve digestion by bringing more blood into the abdominal region. This warming property, and the fact that they can easily be stored in a cold cellar through the winter, makes them an ideal food for the colder months of the year. Moreover, in autumn and winter, they are less expensive than vegetables grown elsewhere and sold out of season.

Ground Vegetables

Nutritionally, ground vegetables such as squash and cabbage fall between the leafy greens and the root vegetables. Like the roots, they are a good source of vitamins and minerals and an excellent supplier of complex carbohydrates. Ground vegetables are good in winter, as they are both warming and filling. In addition, they can satisfy even the sweetest tooth when they are picked ripe and cooked properly.

Vegetables to Avoid

Some vegetables containing irritants and mildly toxic alkaloids (alkaline substances) are listed in Table 7.2 under the heading *To Be Avoided.* Almost all of these have their origin in the tropics. Tomatoes, asparagus, red chard, beet greens, spinach, and rhubarb are also high in oxalic add, which inhibits the absorption of calcium in the body.

Other vegetables, including zucchini, avocado, eggplant, potato, and various edible weeds, are best avoided because they can have an unhealthful acidifying effect on the blood if they are consumed on a regular basis, especially by those living in the temperate zone.

BEANS AND SEA VEGETABLES

Nutritious Food from the Sea

Extracts of marine algae (sea vegetables) are found in almost every type of prepared food, from ice cream and pudding to salad dressings, cheeses, and bread. In fact, any food item that utilizes thickeners or stabilizers probably contains carrageenan, algin, or agar—all extracts of sea vegetables. However, eating sea vegetables in the form of additives is worlds away from eating them directly from the sea.

Table 7.2 Vegetables

FOR REGULAR USE		
Leafy Vegetables	**Ground Vegetables**	**Stem/Root Vegetables**
Bok choy	Acorn squash	Burdock
Broccoli	Buttercup squash	Carrots
Brussels sprouts	Butternut squash	Daikon
Carrot tops	Cabbage	Dandelion root
Chinese cabbage	Cauliflower	Lotus root
Chives	Hubbard squash	Parsnips
Collard greens	Hokkaido pumpkin	Radishes
Daikon greens	Pumpkin	Rutabagas
Dandelion greens		Salsify
Green cabbage		Turnips
Kale		
Leeks		
Mustard greens		
Parsley		
Radish greens		
Scallions		
Turnip greens		
Watercress		
FOR OCCASIONAL USE		
Alfalfa sprouts	Green peas	Romaine lettuce
Bamboo shoots	Iceberg lettuce	Shiitake mushrooms
Bean sprouts	Jerusalem artichokes	Snow peas
Beets	Jinenjo (mountain	String beans
Celery	potatoes)	Summer squash
Corn on the cob	Kohlrabi and greens	Swiss chard
Cucumbers	Mushrooms	Water chestnuts
Endive	Patty pan squash	Yellow wax beans
Escarole	Red cabbage	
TO BE AVOIDED		
Asparagus	Plaintain	Spinach
Avocados	Potatoes	Sweet potatoes
Curly dock	Purslane	Taro (albi)
Eggplant	Red chard	Tomatoes
Fennel	Red peppers	Yams
Ferns	Shepherd's purse	Zucchini
Green peppers	Sorrel	

For centuries, people all over the world have harvested sea vegetables for use as food. The Chinese, Irish, British, Icelanders, Canadians, Japanese, American Indians, Hawaiians, Koreans, Russians, Inuits, and South Africans are just a few of the peoples who have traditionally eaten sea vegetables.

Years ago, in Boston, the purple-colored sea vegetable dulse was sold by street vendors. In the maritime provinces of Canada and in Scotland, a thin, crisp snack made from dulse is still served in pubs. Russians sell a fermented beverage made from sea vegetables and a canned vegetable combination called sea cabbage, which includes vegetables such as beets and tomatoes along with sea vegetables. The coastal Irish have used Irish moss and other sea vegetables for centuries in traditional recipes for breads, pastries, beverages, and gelatins. The Japanese, who probably eat more sea vegetables than any other people, grade their sea vegetables for quality, just as the United States Department of Agriculture grades meat and dairy products.

Sea vegetables are an important component of the macrobiotic diet. As a group, they are among the most nutritious foods on earth. For instance, compared with garden vegetables, kelp has 150 times more iodine and 8 times more magnesium. Dulse is 30 times richer in potassium than bananas are and has 200 times the potency of beets when it comes to iron content. Nori, a brown sea vegetable that is sold in thin rectangular sheets, rivals carrots as a source of vitamin A and has twice the protein of some meats. Hijiki, a blue-black spaghettilike sea vegetable, contains 14 times more calcium than whole milk. Kombu, a brown-colored sea vegetable sold in strips about

Table 7.3 Sea Vegetables

RECOMMENDED

Agar-agar	Hijiki	Kombu
Arame	Irish moss	Nori (laver)
Dulse	Kelp	Wakame

twelve inches long, equals sweet corn in phosphorus. Sea vegetables contain vitamins A, B_1 (thiamine), C, and E, plus the all-important vitamin B_{12}, an essential compound that is rare in vegetarian diets but is needed by the body for healthy neuromuscular function and blood rich in iron.

As they grow, sea vegetables convert the inorganic minerals in seawater into organic mineral salts that are combined with amino acids—the ideal way for us to get the minerals needed to protect the heart and nourish the hair, nails, skin, blood, muscles, and bones. In fact, since the advent of modern farming techniques and the subsequent decline in the quality of topsoil, including sea vegetables in the diet may be the only way we can ensure a healthy supply of trace elements from food. Along with the essential minerals discussed in Chapter 6, trace elements such as cobalt, copper, chromium, fluorine, manganese, molybdenum, selenium, and zinc are needed in small amounts to maintain normal metabolic processes in the body.

Sea vegetables work directly on the blood, alkalizing it if it is too acid and reducing any excess fat or mucus. A substance called alginic acid, found in the darker sea vegetables such as kombu and wakame, transforms toxic metals in the intestines into harmless salts that are easily eliminated. A 1964 study conducted at McGill University in Montreal demonstrated the ability of sea vegetables to remove radioactive strontium 90 from the body.

Beyond their obvious healthfulness, sea vegetables can be quite tasty. Newcomers to the macrobiotic diet will find that when sea vegetables are added to soups and bean dishes, or cooked with fresh vegetables as recommended in the recipes in this book, they accentuate the flavor of the other ingredients.

Beans and Bean Products

For 8,000 years, beans (legumes) have been held in high esteem by cultures all over the world. Since the agricultural revolution of the 1800s, however, they have become less popular in the West, where meat, poultry, and other animal foods have become the primary sources of protein.

Macrobiotics returns the long-neglected bean to its rightful place on the modern dinner table—along with whole grains. Traditional grain-based diets from all over the world have combined grains with beans. In much of Europe, South and Central America, Africa, parts of Asia, and the Middle East, beans and grains are the main sources of protein and carbohydrates.

Modern science has uncovered the reason why this combination works so well: Beans and grains are complementary proteins, one providing the amino acids lacking in the other. Together, these foods supply most of the protein in the macrobiotic diet.

Since beans are particularly rich in high-quality proteins—that is, proteins that are of vegetable origin, are easy for the body to digest and use, and are supplied without saturated animal fats—they are more healthful than meat. In fact, beans replace meat in most vegetarian meat substitutes and in many infant formulas. Moreover, beans (especially after they are sprouted) also contain fairly good supplies of some vitamins and minerals. Table 7.4 lists some of the beans and bean products that are used in the macrobiotic diet.

Whereas whole grains function primarily to provide ready energy in the diet, they are also an important source of the amino acids lacking in beans

Table 7.4 Beans and Bean Products

FOR REGULAR USE		FOR OCCASIONAL USE	
Adzuki beans	Bean sprouts	Lima beans	Red lentils
Chickpeas	Black beans	Navy beans	Soybeans
Lentils, green or brown	Black turtle beans	Peas, dried, whole	Soybeans, black
Miso	Great Northern	Pinto beans	Split peas
Natto (fermented soybeans)	beans		
Tamari (natural soy sauce)	Kidney beans		
Tempeh			
Tofu (soybean curd)			

and bean products. The protein supplied by whole grains is high in quality as well.

Soybeans and Soyfoods

While soybeans are higher in fat and protein than any other beans, they are also the most difficult to digest due to an enzyme called trypsin inhibitor. Soaking, cooking, and fermenting soybeans destroys their trypsin inhibitors, and it is for this reason that these nutritious beans are processed into tofu, natto, tempeh, miso, and the other soyfoods available in natural foods stores.

A major advantage that fermented soyfoods such as tofu and tempeh have over plain-cooked beans and other protein foods are soyfoods' easy-to-digest, quality proteins. Soyfoods are also easy to cook with and taste great in a variety of ways.

The most frequently used soyfoods on the macrobiotic diet are tofu, dried tofu, tempeh, miso, and natural tamari soy sauce. Tofu is processed from soybeans and pressed into cakes. It has served as an important source of protein for more than 2,000 years in China, and more than 1,000 years in Japan. It contains a higher percentage of usable protein than chicken. Tempeh (pronounced TEM-pay) consists of soybeans and/or grains bound by a dense white mold and formed into compact cakes. Like tofu, it is high in protein and low in fat, contains no cholesterol, and has few calories. It is a wonderful food for dieters. In addition, tempeh is one of the richest vegetarian sources of vitamin B_{12}. (Miso and natural tamari soy sauce will be discussed more fully in the next chapter.)

Macrobiotics has promoted the use of traditional soy products in the United States. Their current popularity is due in part to America's increasing consciousness of the relationship between diet and health. Nevertheless, while they provide a relatively inexpensive, tasty supply of excellent-quality and versatile protein, it is important for us to remember that soyfoods aren't a panacea for nutritional problems in this country or for world hunger. They are just one element in a wholesome balanced diet. Like any other high-protein food, they should be eaten in moderation.

We need only small amounts of beans and soyfoods at each meal. The ideal ratio between grains and vegetables on the one hand and beans on the other is seven to one. That is, it is best to eat seven times more whole grains and vegetables than beans and bean products. This translates into about four to six ounces of beans or bean products per day.

Soymilk, soy ice cream, soy yogurt, soy mayonnaise, soy cheesecake, and other soyfoods are not recommended for everyday consumption on the macrobiotic diet. However, they do make good supplementary foods for children or others who are in the process of switching to a more macrobiotic diet.

ORGANICALLY GROWN FOODS

Organic growers do not use synthetically compounded fertilizers, pesticides, herbicides, or fungicides. Instead, they rely on crop rotation, manure, composting of crop residues, and a number of biologically safe measures to control insects, weeds, and other pests. Organically grown foods are more balanced foods, grown on more naturally balanced soil. This balance fosters healthy, balanced people.

EIGHT

Supplementary Macrobiotic Foods

In the macrobiotic diet, condiments and seasonings have greater subtlety than they do in typical modern fare. Condiments and seasonings add color, flavor, and nutrients to macrobiotic foods, as well as improve their digestibility. Because of their varied significance, condiments and seasonings are considered supplementary foods in the macrobiotic diet. Other supplementary foods include fish and seafood, fruits, beverages, and snacks. Cooking ingredients such as natural sweeteners and unrefined oils are also supplementary foods.

While whole grains, beans, and vegetables are the main components of the macrobiotic diet, the supplementary foods play a major role in the overall balance of the diet and its adaptability to individual needs.

CONDIMENTS AND SEASONINGS

The proper use of condiments and seasonings is an important aspect of the macrobiotic diet. Seasonings, for use in cooking, and condiments, for table use, are always employed moderately. Table 8.1 lists the various types that are recommended. Because macrobiotic recipes call for certain regular-use seasonings and condiments quite often, we will briefly discuss their properties and uses.

Sea Salt

Most people today use too much salt, perhaps in an unconscious attempt to compensate for the poor nutritional quality of the salt that is widely available, and to counterbalance a high intake of animal protein and fat. The increased consumption of common salt has led to numerous health problems among the general public. If sea salt is used instead of common salt, however, we find that the body becomes stronger and more balanced, and that there are fewer health problems. In macrobiotics, the quality of salt in the diet is as important as the quantity.

Common salt—the salt used in most prepared foods and eaten by most people in this country—is mined from inland salt deposits, heated to extremely high temperatures, and refined. Potassium iodide or sodium iodide is added to common salt to create iodized salt. Dextrose (sugar), sodium bicarbonate, and sodium silicoaluminate are often added to keep the salt white and easy to pour.

Sea salt is obtained by the simple process of concentrating seawater under the sun. It contains more trace minerals than common salt and no additives. Up to 5 percent of sea salt is composed of naturally occurring potassium, calcium, magnesium, and trace elements, which are responsible for the mild flavor and good taste of sea salt. Most important, these naturally occurring minerals and trace elements can be readily assimilated by the body.

Deciding on the amount of salt to use can be difficult. Depending upon where you live and how much sodium you lose through perspiration, your need for salt will vary. In general, individuals in hotter climates have a slightly greater need for salt, along with an increased need for liquids and unrefined vegetable oils in the diet.

Sea salt is best used in cooking, rather than on the table, because it dissolves more quickly with heat. Gomashio (crushed, toasted sesame seeds mixed with sea salt) is better for table use; the oils, flavor, and minerals in the sesame seeds help balance the raw salt.

The amount of salt in the diet also comes from other condiments, such as natural tamari soy sauce and miso, which are about 20 percent good-quality salt.

Miso, Tamari, and Tamari Soy Sauce

Miso is fermented soybean paste made from soybeans, sea salt, and, sometimes, combinations of whole grains, seasonings, or sea vegetables. Miso is available in many different colors and degrees of saltiness. In addition to being a good source of sodium, it is an excellent source of easily digested protein. In general, miso is rich in live enzymes that aid digestion and promote bowel health.

Good-quality miso that has been naturally fermented is an important ingredient in many recipes, especially soups. It can also be used in bean dishes, salad dressings, condiments, and gravies.

Among natural foods shoppers there remains some confusion between real tamari and tamari soy sauce. Real tamari isn't soy sauce at all, but rather the liquid drained off in the process of making miso. A small amount of real tamari can be used on occasion in place of tamari soy sauce. Real tamari is thicker and stronger in color and flavor, and is slightly more expensive than tamari soy sauce.

Tamari soy sauce is made from soybeans and wheat, without additives or preservatives. Like miso, real tamari and tamari soy sauce are salty-tasting and flavorful. Make sure that the tamari soy sauce you buy is natural, as the ordinary soy sauce sold in supermarkets and many Oriental groceries, and served in restaurants, generally contains corn syrup, artificial coloring, and preservatives.

Brown Rice Vinegar

Brown rice vinegar is simply vinegar made from brown rice. It is used to make salad dressings and relishes. Brown rice vinegar is preferred over wine or cider vinegar because it is less acidic. Nevertheless, it is best to use it in small amounts for flavoring.

Umeboshi

Umeboshi plums are plums pickled in sea salt. These mildly sour and very salty plums may be used whole or in the form of a paste, in cooking or at the table. Umeboshi are highly alkalizing and are used to combat overacidity and stomach upset. They aid in the digestion of foods and promote healthy intestinal flora, as the lactic acid in them is able to neutralize harmful microorganisms. Umeboshi are also helpful in clearing the bowel of putrefaction, thereby reducing gas pains.

Gomashio

Gomashio, or sesame salt, is used as a table condiment. It is made by grinding one part sea salt with ten to sixteen parts toasted whole brown sesame seeds. A mortar and pestle or a Japanese suribachi (a special type of bowl) works well for making sesame salt at home. It can also be purchased in some natural foods stores. A pinch or two of gomashio on whole grains or vegetables will add to their flavor and digestibility.

Table 8.1 Condiments and Seasonings

FOR REGULAR USE		
Brown rice vinegar	Miso	Sauerkraut
Ginger	Mustard, natural	Scallions
Gomashio	Nori condiment	Sea salt
Daikon, grated	Onions	Tamari (natural soy sauce)
Horseradish	Parsley	Tekka
Kelp-sesame salt	Pickled vegetables	Umeboshi plums or paste
Kombu condiment	Roasted sea vegetable	Umeboshi vinegar
Mirin	powder	

TO BE AVOIDED		
All unnatural, artificial, and/or	Ginseng	Spices (curry, pepper, cumin, chili, etc.)
chemically processed seasonings	Gray sea salt	Wine
Apple cider vinegar	Iodized salt	Wine vinegar
Commercial soy sauce	Mayonnaise	
Common salt	Soy margarine	

A Note on Spices

One important point to remember about the macrobiotic diet is that the foods themselves, enhanced with just a little sea salt, flavor the meals. Black pepper, catsup, mustard, and strong spices, such as cayenne pepper, turmeric, cumin, and curry powder, overpower delicately flavored meals and are generally not used in macrobiotic cooking. It is generally best to avoid stimulants (such as ginseng) and aromatic herbs, although they may be used in cooking for special occasions.

NATURAL SWEETENERS

All sweeteners are concentrated sugars, and if abused, they tend to affect blood sugar levels and overall health. Sweeteners aren't particularly recom-

Table 8.2 Natural Sweeteners

FOR OCCASIONAL USE		
Amasake	Fruits, dried (temperate-climate)	Raisins
Apple juice or cider	Fruits, fresh or cooked	Rice malt
Barley malt	Mirin	Yinnie (rice) syrup
Chestnuts		

mended as a source of nutrition, but moderate amounts of good-quality, natural fruit and vegetable sweeteners are not harmful. Honey, molasses, and so-called "natural sugar" ought to be avoided along with cane and beet sugar (sucrose). The best sweeteners to use are rice syrup and barley malt, which are both made by cooking down grains.

Amasake (rice milk) is a sweetener made by cooking sweet rice and then adding koji, a fermentation starter. After a few hours of fermentation, the rice is cooked again. Mixed with water, amasake can make a sweet milk substitute or a delicious pudding. It can also be cooked down to make a syrup for sweetening other foods. Regardless of the climate or geographical location, all of the natural sweeteners listed in Table 8.2 can be used moderately.

UNREFINED COOKING OILS

The oils used in macrobiotic cooking are unrefined, unlike commercial oils. Commercial corn oil, for example, is processed by cooking corn in water at a high temperature and then crushing it and treating it with lye and bleach. The oil is reheated in a vacuum for twelve hours to deodorize it. Finally, a synthetic antioxidant is added to prevent spoilage. To make margarine, the refined oil is saturated with hydrogen to solidify it. This processing results in inferior-quality fats, which are difficult to digest.

Naturally extracted, unrefined vegetable oils are easier to digest. They also strengthen cell and capillary structure, lubricate the skin and hair, and provide raw materials for the production of lecithin, which plays an important role in lowering blood cholesterol levels. In addition, unrefined vegetable oils contain a natural preservative in the form of vitamin E.

While a deficiency of fats is virtually impossible on the macrobiotic diet, since most natural foods contain some fat, a shortage of essential fatty acids can lead to cold hands and feet, stunted growth in children, dermatitis, poor sexual performance, hot flashes, and a lowered resistance to stresses of all kinds. Over the long run, too few fats in the diet could also damage the nervous system.

Oil is similar to salt in that while a moderate amount is necessary, a lot can be harmful. A teaspoon of oil per person, used every day or every other day (in cooking) is usually adequate.

Two specific unrefined oils recommended for regular use are corn and sesame oil (light or dark). These are chemically stable and tolerate heat well. Besides corn and sesame oils, small amounts of unrefined sunflower, safflower, soybean, olive, and peanut oils can be used. As Table 8.3 indicates, you should avoid the use of cottonseed oil, palm kernel oil, and cocoa butter (oil made from coconuts). These are less stable and become rancid more easily. Many so-called health-food candies, such as the popular carob treats,

Table 8.3 Cooking Oils

FOR REGULAR USE		
Corn oil	Sesame oil, light and dark	
FOR OCCASIONAL USE		
Olive oil	Safflower oil	Sunflower oil
Peanut oil	Soybean oil	
TO BE AVOIDED		
Butter, lard, and other animal fats	Vegetable shortening	Soy margarine
Margarine	Refined or chemically processed oils	

often use these inferior oils because they are highly saturated and simulate the texture of chocolate.

FRESH FISH AND SEAFOODS

The macrobiotic diet for people living in temperate (four-season) climates need not be totally vegetarian; it can include moderate amounts of white-meat fish and certain shellfish. Besides being exposed to fewer chemicals and pollutants than other animal protein sources, fish is nutritionally superior.

Livestock and other animal protein sources cannot be compared with the wild game our ancestors ate because today's animals are fed hormones and antibiotics to artificially fatten them for market. They are also given shelter from the elements and all the food they can eat. This means fattier meat and poorer-quality milk. Not only did our ancestors consume a smaller amount of animal proteins and fats than we do, but what they did eat was better for them.

Meats are often aged for months, and preservatives and red dyes are used to prevent them from turning black and blue. Poultry is also injected with preservatives and dipped in solutions to increase shelf life. Fresh fish, especially freshwater or ocean fish caught locally, is usually eaten within two or three days of the catch. It is generally marketed without added hormones, coloring agents, antibiotics, or preservatives. One exception is freshwater fish (especially trout) bred in fish farms, as they have been fed an unnatural diet and raised in an artificial environment.

Most fish is lower in fat and cholesterol than red meats, milk, eggs, cheese, yogurt, or poultry, and it is generally higher in its percentage of usable protein than any of these as well. It is also easier to digest.

When eating fish, it is a good idea to increase the amount of vegetables at the meal, especially greens. It is also good to use a garnish such as several tablespoons of grated raw daikon with a few drops of tamari. This will help to balance the nutrients in the fish and aid in its digestion.

Since they are higher in fat and cholesterol, shellfish should be used less

Table 8.4 Fresh Fish and Seafoods

FOR REGULAR USE

Flounder	Herring	Trout
Haddock	Smelt	
Halibut	Sole	

FOR OCCASIONAL USE

Carp	Red snapper	Oysters
Clams	Scrod	
Cod	Shrimp	

TO BE AVOIDED

Bluefish	Swordfish	Other fishes with red meat or blue skin
Mackerel	Tuna	
Salmon		

often than white-meat fish. Individual servings of fish and shellfish can be about four to six ounces, eaten one or two times per week (if you are in good health). As supplementary foods, fish and shellfish enhance the macrobiotic diet, but they are not necessary for balanced nutrition. Table 8.4 lists the varieties of fresh fish and seafoods that are used, along with the types that are best avoided.

When you shop for fish, find out when and where it was caught. Whenever possible, follow the reports of water quality in your area, and do not buy any fish or shellfish, including freshwater fish, from polluted or contaminated waters.

MACROBIOTIC SNACKS

Snacks are especially good between meals if you are hungry. There are many tasty natural snacks to choose from.

Table 8.5 Snacks

FOR OCCASIONAL USE		
Almonds	Popcorn, homemade	Sesame seeds
Chestnuts	Pumpkin seeds	Sunflower seeds
Peanuts	Rice cakes	Walnuts
Pecans	Roasted grains and beans	

TO BE AVOIDED		
Brazil nuts	Filberts (hazelnuts)	Pistachios
Cashew nuts	Macadamia nuts	

Roasted seeds and nuts, lightly salted with sea salt or natural tamari soy sauce, make a delightful snack. As they are rich in fat and somewhat difficult to digest, it is best to eat them in small amounts. It is most healthful to limit the use of roasted seeds and nuts to two or three handfuls a week as a snack, with only a small amount more, if desired, used as an ingredient in preparing breads, desserts, or vegetable and grain dishes. Small quantities of nut or seed butters (such as sesame, sunflower, or natural peanut butter) can also be used occasionally.

As Table 8.5 indicates, some other good snacks include rice cakes, popcorn, and the roasted grains and beans available at natural foods stores.

FRESH AND DRIED FRUITS

Fresh fruit is a delicious addition to the macrobiotic diet. Fruits that are unripe, those grown out of season and shipped to the winter zone, and tropical fruits are not recommended for people living in the temperate climate zone. However, a healthy individual living in a tropical area may use small amounts of tropical fruits as they become available in season. Table 8.6 shows the various temperate and tropical climate fruits.

Table 8.6 Fresh and Dried Fruits

TEMPERATE CLIMATE FRUITS (GENERALLY FOR OCCASIONAL USE)

Apples	Currants	Raspberries
Apricots	Grapes	Raisins
Blackberries	Honeydew melon	Strawberries
Blueberries	Peaches	Tangerines
Cantaloupe	Pears	Watermelon
Cherries	Plums	
Cranberries	Prunes	

TROPICAL FRUITS AND JUICES (GENERALLY TO BE AVOIDED)

Avocados	Grapefruits	Mangoes
Bananas	Guavas	Oranges
Coconuts	Kiwis	Papayas
Dates	Lemons	Pineapples
Figs	Limes	

Fruits that have been sprayed or chemically treated in any way are best avoided. Locally grown, unsprayed fruits (in season), and dried fruits such as raisins, prunes, apples, pears, apricots, cherries, and currants are recommended. These are best eaten cooked (with a pinch of sea salt if desired) or dried. Upon occasion, fresh, uncooked fruits may be eaten. Since so many fruits are picked unripe, sold out of season, or sprayed with pesticides, it is best to limit fruit consumption to a few servings per week.

BEVERAGES

The beverages most commonly consumed in America are soft drinks, orange juice, tea, coffee, beer, wine, whiskey, and milk. Many of these have been linked to a number of health problems. Tea, coffee, and colas have been implicated for their caffeine content; flavored soft drinks and juices for their sugar and additives; orange juice due to its acidity and allergic reactions reported by users; commercial beers and alcoholic beverages for their additives, preservatives, and alcohol; and milk for its cholesterol and fat. In place of these drinks, the macrobiotic diet uses a variety of special teas, coffee substitutes, and occasionally fresh juices and other beverages. These are listed in Table 8.7.

Tea, especially twig or stem (bancha) tea, is a healthful and satisfying beverage that can be enjoyed warm or cool. Many varieties of tea, including bancha, come from the plant known botanically as *Camellia sinensis,* which is cultivated in different parts of the world. But teas from this plant vary widely. When and where the plants are grown and harvested, and which parts of the plant are used, determine the strength and caffeine content of

Table 8.7 Beverages

FOR REGULAR USE		
Amasake	Roasted barley tea	Spring or well water
Bancha tea	Roasted rice tea	

FOR OCCASIONAL USE		
Dandelion tea	Kombu tea	Mu tea
Grain coffee		

FOR LESS FREQUENT USE		
Apple juice or cider	Green tea	Seed and nut milks
Barley green tea	Naturally fermented beer	Vegetable juices
Fruit (temperate-climate) juices	Sake (rice wine)	

TO BE AVOIDED		
Alcohol	Commercial beers	Juice drinks, commercial
Artificially flavored beverages	Decaffeinated coffee	Municipal or tap water
Black tea	Distilled water	Soft drinks
Coffee	Herbal teas (mint, rose hips, etc.)	Wine

the tea. Teas made from young leaves and buds (sold in many gourmet shops) are the most stimulating. Next comes black teas, the most commonly used teas. Both of these types are too stimulating for daily use.

The teas used on the macrobiotic diet are different. Whereas some of them may contain minute quantities of caffeine, they are not processed to increase their caffeine content. Processed brands, which are high in caffeine, are best avoided.

Other teas (not made from the tea plant) recommended for use on the macrobiotic diet are roasted barley or rice tea, dandelion root tea, kombu tea (from kombu sea vegetable), and umeboshi tea (from salted plums). In addition, you may use mu tea, which is an especially strengthening blend of traditional non-stimulating herbs. Other aromatic or medicinal herb teas, such as peppermint, rose hips, or chamomile are not recommended. Herbs should be treated as medicine; to use them indiscriminately could be harmful.

All of the beverages mentioned above can be used as a substitute for coffee, but if a more robust flavor is desired, grain coffee made from a blend of roasted grains (with or without chicory root) can be used on occasion. All hot teas and beverages are best made with pure spring or well water, as municipal water supplies may be contaminated with harmful substances such as chlorine or sodium fluoride.

USING SUPPLEMENTARY FOODS

Supplementary foods may make up as much as 10 percent of the macrobiotic diet, depending upon your individual tastes and nutritional needs. As a group, the supplementary foods are the most flexible part of the diet. In Chapter 10, we will discuss some of the ways in which the diet may be modified.

If you have specific questions regarding modifications of the standard diet, you may wish to seek the guidance of an experienced macrobiotic counselor; however, in general, if you are in good overall health, you may enjoy moderate amounts of the supplementary foods discussed in this chapter.

NINE

Yin and Yang

Everything in the universe is constantly changing. Each day we experience the result of this unceasing motion as night changes into day, activity changes into rest, youth into old age, life into death, and death into rebirth. An understanding of the changes that govern our lives and the natural environment, and a recognition of the interrelationship between opposite yet complementary tendencies within these changes, helps us to achieve harmony in our bodies and minds.

The principle of yin and yang is the philosophical foundation of macrobiotics. The way to practice this universal principle in daily life was taught by Lao Tzu, Confucius, Buddha, Moses, Jesus, Muhammad, and other great teachers throughout history. To understand this simple principle and then to live its basic laws is the greatest way to perfect health and long life.

The principle of yin and yang is also known as the "unifying principle" because it states that antagonistic forces complement and unify each other. A clear example of this is man and woman. Though men and women are opposites in many ways, they depend on each other for continued existence. Together, they form a unity, each acquiring aspects of the other.

Many different interpretations have been given to yin and yang throughout history. Several thousand years ago in China, for example, the universal process of change was called the Tao. The Taoists and others based their teachings on the underlying principle of yin and yang. In the Hindu religion, Brahma, the absolute, becomes Shiva and Parvati, the god and goddess whose cosmic dance gives rise to all phenomena in the universe. Similarly, in the Shinto religion, Ame-no-Minakanushi, who stands for infinity, becomes Takami-musubi and Kami-musubi, the gods of centrifugality and centripetality, respectively, from whom the phenomenal universe arises.

In the West, the underlying principle of yin and yang has been expressed in countless ways by various philosophers and teachers. For example, the ancient Greek philosopher Empedocles viewed the universe as an eternal playground of two opposite, yet complementary forces, which he called love and strife. Another classical philosopher, Heraclitus, referring to the eternal process of change as Logos, taught of the opposite, yet complementary nature of all phenomena.

In Judaism, the principle of complementary opposites is expressed in the symbol of the six-pointed Star of David, showing the balanced intersection of descending and ascending triangles. More recently, key ideas in the works of writers and philosophers such as Ralph Waldo Emerson, Henry David Thoreau, Georg Wilhelm Friedrich Hegel, and Walter Russell have expressed the underlying principle of yin and yang, while a more natural way of life, based on balance, has been advocated by many thinkers, including Edward Carpenter, Samuel Butler, and George Bernard Shaw.

YIN AND YANG IN MACROBIOTICS

Macrobiotics focuses on the dynamics of yin and yang in daily life. Yin is the name given to energy or movement that has a centrifugal, or outward, direc-

Table 9.1 Examples of Yin and Yang

CHARACTERISTIC	YIN (∇)	YANG ($\triangle$)
Atomic particle	Electron	Proton
Attitude	More gentle, passive	More aggressive, active
Biological	More vegetable quality	More animal quality
Climate	Temperate, colder	Tropical, warmer
Direction	Ascent; vertical; outward	Descent; horizontal; inward
Flavor	Sweet	Salty
Food preparation	Less cooked	More cooked
Form	Longer, thinner	Shorter, thicker
Function	Diffusion	Fusion
Humidity	More wet	More dry
Light	Darker	Brighter
Movement	More inactive; slower	More active; faster
Nerves	Peripheral, orthosympathetic	Central, parasympathetic
Organ structure	More hollow, expansive	More dense, compacted
Position	More outward, peripheral	More inward, central
Sex	Female	Male
Shape	More expansive	More contracted
Size	Larger	Smaller
Temperature	Colder	Hotter
Tendency	Expansion	Contraction
Texture	Softer	Harder
Vibration	Shorter wave, higher frequency	Longer wave, lower frequency
Weight	Lighter	Heavier
Work	More psychological, mental	More physical, social

tion, and results in expansion. Thus diffusion, dispersion, expansion, and separation are all yin tendencies. Yang, on the other hand, denotes energy or movement that has a centripetal, or inward, direction, and results in contraction. Fusion, gathering, contraction, and organization are yang tendencies.

The forces of yin and yang are the most basic and primary, and are found throughout creation. All movement, formation, change, and interaction can be understood in terms of a basic yin and yang equation.

By looking at which of these energies predominates in plants, foods, or individuals, we can classify them as more yin or more yang. However, since all things are relative, nothing is ever completely yin or yang. From an understanding of yin and yang tendencies, we can learn ways to achieve natural harmony and balance in the body and in life.

In the world around us, the sun, daytime, heat, and summer all display yang tendencies, while the moon, night, cold, and winter reflect more yin qualities. In the human body we can see the action of both yin and yang in the expansion and contraction of the lungs and heart, or in the stomach and intestines during digestion. Being active, animals (including humans) are more yang than plants, which are stationary. As Table 9.1 suggests, there are a number of factors that can be used to determine yin or yang qualities.

YIN AND YANG IN FOODS

Watery, cooling yin plant foods grow in hot yang climates. Denser, hardier yang plant foods grow in temperate yin climates. When we begin to realize that our food affects our ability to adapt to local climates and conditions, the importance of balance becomes more clear. All of us follow our natural instincts to some extent in order to maintain balance. When it is cold, we turn up the heat. When it becomes warm, we seek refreshment. The summer brings lighter eating and less cooking, the winter heavier eating and more thorough cooking. Macrobiotics helps us to become more aware of our intuitive needs for foods well suited to our local environment. It also tells us how to cook and prepare these foods in harmony with our immediate needs and conditions.

Red meat, poultry, hard cheeses, and eggs are more yang than plants. They are the result of a concentration of plants eaten by an animal.

A further division into yin and yang characteristics can be made within the plant kingdom itself. A northern pine, for example, has short, hard needles, while the southern pine develops larger, longer, and softer ones. Root vegetables and seeds are more yang than leaves and branches. Above ground vegetables such as winter squashes or pumpkins are more yang—more dense and less watery—than tree fruits. In general, plants that grow quickly in warm climates or hot weather, and those that have a higher water content, are more yin. Tropical fruits like papayas, mangoes, avocados, bananas, and citrus fruits, and tropical vegetables such as potatoes, tomatoes, spinach, zucchini, eggplant, and yams are all yin compared with the more hardy plants of northern origin. In the temperate north, indigenous fruits, grains, vegetables, seeds, beans, and nuts are smaller, grow more slowly, contain less liquid, and are more yang.

Figure 9.1 lists from top (yin) to botton (yang) and right (yin) to left (yang) many foods commonly eaten on the macrobiotic diet and in many parts of the world.

Within each category of foods listed on the chart, there are yin and yang variations. For example, among the grains, buckwheat (the most yang) thrives in cold climates and in the mountains. Corn (the most yin) likes hot summer weather and grows well in the tropics. Brown rice is in between. Relatively small beans such as adzuki are more yang than lima beans and soybeans, which are larger and contain more fat and oil. The same is true for nuts and seeds—the smaller and less oily they are, the more yang. Sesame seeds, which are hard and small, are more yang than larger and more oily Brazil nuts or walnuts. Swordfish, salmon, bluefish, mackerel, or tuna (all faster, larger, and more powerful fish) are more yang than smaller white-meat fish such as flounder or sole. Table 9.2 lists the general yin and yang variations of the foods by food category.

The macrobiotic diet is made up of foods located in the center of Figure 9.1: the foods that are most balanced in terms of yin and yang and in nutritional factors for adults in a temperate climate. (The practical application of the workings of yin and yang in cooking and eating will be discussed in Chapter 10.) When we eat foods out of harmony with our bodily needs, such as meats, eggs, and hard salty cheeses (all yang), we create an equal and opposite craving for sugar; strong or stimulating spices, herbs, or condi-

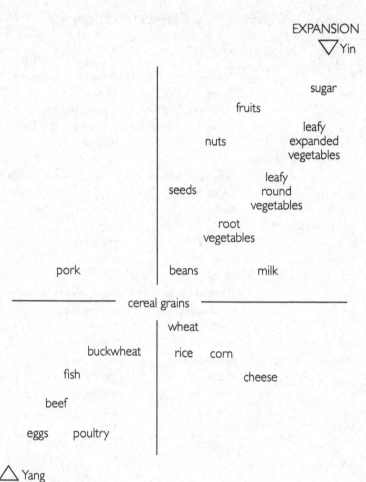

EXPANSION
∇ Yin

sugar

fruits

nuts

leafy
expanded
vegetables

seeds

leafy
round
vegetables

root
vegetables

pork   beans   milk

——————— cereal grains ———————

wheat

buckwheat   rice   corn

fish   cheese

beef

eggs   poultry

△ Yang
CONTRACTION

Figure 9.1   General Yin (∇) and Yang (△)
Categorizations of Foods

Table 9.2 Variations in Yin and Yang by Food Category

	CATEGORY	(△) YANG	(▽) YIN
Yin	Sugar	Raw	Refined
	Fruits	Smaller	Larger
		Growing on the ground	Growing on a tree
		Grown in a colder climate	Grown in a warmer climate
	Nuts	Less oily	More oily
	Leafy expanded vegetables	Smaller	Larger
		Grown in a colder climate	Grown in a warmer climate
	Seeds	Smaller	Larger
	Leafy round vegetables	Smaller	Larger
	Root vegetables	Smaller	Larger
	Pork	Less fatty	More fatty
	Beans (legumes)	Small	Large
	Milk	Less fatty	More fatty
	Cereal grains	Grown in a colder climate	Grown in a warmer climate
	Fish	Faster-moving	Slower-moving
		Smaller	Larger
	Beef	Drier	More fatty
	Cheese	More condensed	Less condensed
		Less fatty	More fatty
		Saltier	Sweeter
	Eggs	Smaller	Larger
	Poultry	Smaller	Larger
Yang		High-flying	Low-flying

ments; coffee; alcohol; ice cream; and tropical fruits; (all yin), in an attempt to balance our physical and mental condition. The swings from one extreme to the other can destroy the foundation of good health and lead to disease.

All physical and mental imbalances can be explained as being caused by excessive yin, excessive yang, or a combination of excessive yin and yang in food choice, attitude, and lifestyle. An example of a symptom arising from excess yin is a headache caused when the cells and tissues of the brain expand due to an overindulgence in alcohol. A headache caused by excess yang, on the other hand, arises when the cells and tissues of the brain contract and press against one another, causing pain. This example shows that seemingly similar symptoms can arise from opposite causes. It also explains why aspirin (extreme yin) can relieve some headaches (ones due to yang causes), while it is powerless to relieve a headache due to a hangover (an excess yin cause).

Many factors are weighed by the trained macrobiotic counselor in determining a person's overall condition and the best diet for that person. Nevertheless, the macrobiotic diet for healing usually involves a combination of whole grains, vegetables, beans, and supplementary foods—the standard diet outlined in this book—adapted to suit the individual's needs.

Beyond the purely physical effects of extreme yin or yang foods and lifestyles, these imbalances have a profound impact on a person's psyche as well.

THE BIGGER THE FRONT, THE BIGGER THE BACK

In everything there is a front and a back. Macrobiotic theory suggests that the bigger the front, the bigger the back will be. For example, the huge military arms race and its implications for the future survival of human life (the front) have also created a global desire for world peace (the back). Modern society's tendency to take a symptomatic approach to illness (the front) has created an inspiring revolution in health care called the holistic approach (the back). Our sedentary lifestyle and questionable habits (the front) have created a rapidly expanding natural foods industry spurred by people interested in improving the quality of our nutrition, and a widespread interest in fitness (the back). This is another illustration of the principle of balance like that which underlies the macrobiotic diet and lifestyle.

TEN

Balancing the Macrobiotic Diet

In addition to foods high in complex carbohydrates, fiber, vitamins, and minerals, we need a balanced diet. Correct balancing of the macrobiotic diet promotes harmony between the immediate environment and the body, and allows for flexibility in designing a diet that best suits personal nutritional requirements.

As we discussed in Chapter 1, eating locally grown foods is fundamental to the macrobiotic way. Locally grown foods help the body to adapt to seasonal changes, thus preventing seasonal imbalances such as colds or flu, as well as more serious illnesses. There are other important advantages to eating local foods, not the least of which is a cooler body in the heat and a warmer one in the cold.

The human body expands in heat and contracts in cold. A warm bath, for example, soothes and relaxes (expands) tight muscles, whereas a cold bath stimulates and invigorates (contracts) them. During summer, a wristwatch fits more tightly as a result of expansion of the body, while in winter it fits more loosely. The summer season, which is yang, creates a more yin (expanded) body condition. Winter creates the reverse. The food we eat affects the expansion and contraction of the body as well.

During summer we tend to eat more yin foods and use lighter cooking for balance. We emphasize foods rich in vitamin C, especially garden vegetables, along with summer grains such as corn, which have an expansive effect on the body and keep us cool. After the autumn harvest, the transition to the yin season (winter) begins. With it, the body becomes more yang (contracted). To encourage the change, we eat more yang vegetables such as winter squashes, root vegetables, cabbage, and hardy greens, and autumn grains such as oats, wheat, and buckwheat. We also increase the amount of fats and protein foods such as beans (legumes) and white-meat fish. These foods, coupled with longer cooking times, keep the body warmer and more comfortable during winter.

While it is best to select fresh foods from your immediate locality, you may use other foods brought in from greater distances. In general, more perishable items are best when harvested locally; more readily storable foods, such as grains, beans, sea vegetables, and sea salt need not be of local origin. Table 10.1 below provides some guidelines for determining the ideal geographic ranges for foods and ingredients imported to your area.

THE ADAPTABILITY OF THE MACROBIOTIC DIET

Within the continental United States, there are differences in climate and environment that you may consider when adapting the macrobiotic diet, and especially cooking styles, to your individual needs.

In the southern portions of the United States, where temperatures can soar over one hundred degrees for days at a time during the summer, lighter eating is appropriate. As previously mentioned, a diet of whole grains, lightly cooked summer garden vegetables, light soups, pressed and raw salads, and some fruit, keeps the body cool and comfortable.

In more northerly or mountainous regions where the climate is cooler,

Table 10.1 Geographic Ranges

FOOD OR INGREDIENT	IDEAL GEOGRAPHIC RANGE
Water	Immediate environment; ideally from a well or clear spring near your home.
Fruit	Same climatic and geographical region; for example, the New England area for someone in Massachusetts or the southern states for someone in Alabama.
Vegetables	More extended area, but similar to the place in which you live; for example, the New England, mid-Atlantic, and midwestern states for someone in New England.
Whole grains and beans (legumes)	Further extended areas that share similar geographical and climatic conditions; for example, anywhere in North America for people living in the United States.
Sea vegetables	Even further extended than the above; generally, anywhere within the same climatic belt; for example, people living in North America or Europe may eat sea vegetables from either place or from temperate zones of the Far East.
Sea salt	The entire hemisphere, either Northern or Southern, depending upon where you live.

and during winter, the macrobiotic diet consists of a greater proportion of hearty foods—beans, seeds, nuts, oils, soyfoods, and fish. Longer cooking times are used to generate more body warmth. In macrobiotic cooking for cooler regions, local apples, pears, or dried fruits stewed or baked into desserts replace the fruits or juices used in warmer areas. Table 10.2 summarizes some key climatic factors and appropriate adjustments.

Table 10.2 Modifications for Climatic Factors

CLIMATIC FACTOR	LOWER	HIGHER
Temperature	More thorough cooking; stronger seasoning	Shorter cooking times; less seasoning
Humidity	More water in cooking	Less water in cooking

BALANCING YIN AND YANG IN THE DIET

Understanding the subtle balancing of foods in the macrobiotic diet in terms of yin and yang is important for personal adaptations of the diet. In general, the modern diet is composed of extreme foods that can cause the body to become simultaneously too yin and too yang. The typical modern diet tends to foster an expanded (or yin) outer appearance of the body, together with inner rigidity and hardness (an overly yang internal state). The most obvious outward sign of this is overweight. Internally, the extreme yang condition is manifested as tense, tight muscles, stiffness in the joints, accumulation of excess fats and water, and hardening of the arteries.

Eating macrobiotically leads to a more yang appearance; the body becomes slimmer, with better muscle definition and more graceful contours. Internally, the body becomes more balanced, functioning more smoothly and efficiently. The overall benefits of this more balanced condition include increased flexibility and capacity for relaxation.

However, if fish and overcooked, excessively salty, relatively yang foods are overemphasized in the diet, the individual may experience strong cravings for yin foods such as ice cream, sugared desserts, or alcoholic beverages. When macrobiotic meals are balanced in terms of yin and yang, cravings for extreme foods are minimized, and the body becomes more fit and flexible gradually, at a natural pace.

Whole grains, which are a major component of the macrobiotic diet, are centrally balanced. That is, they are neither too yin nor too yang. However, since different cooking methods affect the subtle balancing of yin and yang, even in whole grains, it is important to understand the qualities of all the foods on the macrobiotic diet and to select a wide variety of them in your daily meals.

Beans, which are more yin because of their higher protein and fat content, are balanced when cooked with a relatively yang sea vegetable, such as kombu. Vegetables (more yin) are balanced by a little tamari soy sauce or sea salt (more yang). Fruits are also more balanced in terms of yin and yang when they are cooked with a pinch of sea salt.

An afternoon or evening meal that includes miso soup—which, because of its salty taste and high mineral content, is relatively yang—is balanced by the addition of fresh lightly steamed vegetables, a pressed salad or pickled vegetables, and bancha tea (all more yin). A breakfast consisting of miso soup, whole oats, or another whole-grain cereal is balanced by garnishes such as chopped scallions, chopped chives, or toasted nori. Cooked fruit, apple butter, or a few raisins may be used occasionally to balance a breakfast meal.

Fish or seafood (yang) is balanced by the addition of vegetables, such as leafy greens and grated raw daikon, or by garnishes or seasonings such as scallions, ginger, or natural mustard (all more yin). Soba noodles, which are more yang, are balanced by the addition of chopped scallions or a liquid broth.

Desserts made from fresh fruit and whole-grains or whole-grain flour are more yin. When used occasionally, they help to satisfy the natural desire for sweets, while the body becomes more healthy. Ending meals with a small amount of naturally sweet foods such as plain brown rice or bancha tea reduces the craving for desserts. When meals reflect the proper balance of yin and yang, they are flavorful, satisfying, and visually appealing.

ADOPTING THE MACROBIOTIC DIET

Changing the eating habits of a lifetime is quite a challenge, but one well worth the effort. Unless you are in poor health and are being counseled on a regular basis by a qualified macrobiotic counselor, a gradual, yet steady, transition to the macrobiotic diet is best.

Begin by reducing the amount of saturated fats, refined starches, and sugars in your diet. Eat whole grains, vegetables, beans, and sea vegetables more frequently. Always try to avoid foods that are high in cholesterol, saturated fats, sugar, and additives.

It is best to adopt the macrobiotic diet with a confident and unhurried attitude. Begin by adding whole foods such as pressure-cooked brown rice to your present diet, and gradually increase the variety of natural foods and cooking styles you use. Eliminate strong-tasting spices and seasonings, and replace them with appropriate cooking methods that enable the inherent flavor and vitality of natural foods to come through. With the help of the chapters on food preparation and the recipes in this book, you will be well on the way to preparing delectable macrobiotic meals as if you have been doing so all your life. You may also want to attend macrobiotic cooking classes, which are offered in many parts of the United States. (See the Resources section at the end of this book.)

Transitional Foods

As you change your eating habits toward the macrobiotic diet, you can use certain transitional foods as replacements for any of the foods you miss. Table 10.3 lists a number of transitional foods you may find helpful.

When you remove processed and refined food items from your shelves and cupboards, you will be taking the first step toward a more healthful lifestyle.

Some of the foods and ingredients listed in the right-hand column of the table are suggested primarily for use as replacements for the more conventional items listed on the left. They may be of use to you as transitional items during the period of time in which you are becoming familiar with macrobiotic cooking methods and techniques. For example, if you are baking a pie, you may wish to replace the sweetener called for in your favorite recipe with barley malt, yinnie (rice) syrup, or maple syrup. You may also wish to try making the crust with arrowroot or kuzu and whole-wheat pastry flour instead of eggs and bleached white flour. In this way, you may become more sensitive to the natural flavors and qualities of your cooking ingredients. An awareness and appreciation of these properties, among others, is fundamental to the macrobiotic way. It is important to remember, however, that the

Table 10.3 Transitional Foods

Please note that the purpose of this table is to assist you in making the transition to macrobiotics wisely and in an informed way. It does *not* set forth guidelines for daily eating in accordance with macrobiotic principles. Further, it is important to point out that while transitional foods and ingredients resemble the flavor and texture of foods that are typically part of the modern diet, and while they offer some nutritive value in place of empty calories and potentially harmful chemical additives, many of them are *suitable only for very occasional use* in macrobiotic cooking and eating.

FOOD CATEGORY	TYPICAL MODERN FOODS AND INGREDIENTS TO AVOID	TRANSITIONAL FOODS AND INGREDIENTS TO SUBSTITUTE
Baked goods	Items made with dairy products; yeasted and refined items	Homemade popcorn, rice cakes, unyeasted breads, whole-grain desserts, whole grains
Beverages	Alcoholic beverages, coffee, commercial black and herbal teas, processed fruit juices, milk, soft drinks, tap water	Amasake, bancha tea, green tea, mu tea, natural fruit juices, rice wine, seed or nut milk, soymilk, spring or well water
Fats	Butter, cream, cheese, margarine, mayonnaise, milk, yogurt	Nut butter; unrefined corn, olive, peanut, safflower, sesame, soy, sunflower oils
Fruits and sweet vegetables	Canned, with preservatives and/or sugar; dried, with additives; tropical	Carrots, parsnips, squashes; natural dried fruits; temperate-climate fruits
Gelatin	all brands	Agar-agar (kanten)
Protein foods	Beef, cheese, dark-meat fish, lamb, pork, poultry, veal	Beans (legumes), seitan, soyfoods, tofu, white-meat fish, whole grains
Eggs	Common hen's eggs	Arrowroot or kuzu powder (in baking), tofu
Salt	Common (rock) salt, gray sea salt, iodized salt	Gomashio, miso, sea salt, sea vegetable powders, tamari, tekka
Sweeteners	Artificial sweeteners, chocolate, corn syrup, honey, molasses, sugar, fructose	Amasake, apple juice or cider, barley malt, fresh or cooked fruits, maple syrup, mirin, natural dried fruits, yinnie (rice) syrup
White-flour products	All	Whole-wheat or other whole-grain cakes, cereals, cookies, noodles, pies, etc.

use of more healthful ingredients is only one part of a more healthful lifestyle. A variety of cooking techniques and proper food combinations, as discussed throughout this book, are also important. In addition, the macrobiotic way of eating brings the body into harmony with the seasonal changes in our natural environment. The macrobiotic way of life incorporates moderate exercise and a positive philosophy as well as a healthful diet.

The recommendations about the macrobiotic way of eating are not arbitrary, but rather are founded upon the traditional ways of eating shared by many people around the world. Their efficacy has been demonstrated by the general good health and vitality, and in many cases, the recovery from serious illness, of individuals who have adopted this way of eating. The standard macrobiotic dietary recommendations have been developed over many years of study and experience. In addition, trained macrobiotic counselors help individuals to modify the standard diet to suit their particular needs.

All of the dietary recommendations are based upon the proper use of whole, natural foods and are designed to promote balance and health in the body. These qualities and strengths are needed more than ever in our complex modern world.

EATING MACROBIOTICALLY

It is best to eat a large variety of wholesome foods, but it isn't necessary, or even healthful, to eat them all at the same meal. An average macrobiotic meal might consist of a bowl of soup, a dish made from one or two whole grains, a few different cooked vegetables, a bean dish or a small serving of white-meat fish, and perhaps a small salad. Eating macrobiotically means understanding the importance of balance, in both the selection and preparation of foods.

When cooking, use a variety of seasonings, rather than always relying on tamari or sea salt alone for flavor. Also use a variety of cooking styles such as nishime, sautéing, pressure-cooking, boiling, baking, and steaming.

Maintaining the ideal proportions of whole grains, vegetables, beans, and the supplementary foods is important. (Refer again to Figure 1.2 on page 14 for an illustration of this.) Keep in mind, however, that not every meal need be balanced just so; it is more important to balance the foods eaten during the course of the day. For example, if breakfast consists of miso soup, oatmeal, toast with apple butter, and bancha tea (essentially a whole-grain meal), then the lunch and dinner meals ought to include more vegetables and supplementary foods in relation to whole grains. However, it is important to include whole grains at every meal.

Every day, try to use two or three different whole grains; seven or more different vegetables of varied colors, some eaten raw (pickled or pressed) and some cooked; a sea vegetable or two; and at least one kind of bean or soy-food. If you are healthy you may use white-meat fish a few times per week.

Eat at least two, and preferably three, meals each day. If you get hungry between meals, have a snack such as a rice cake. Eat enough food to maintain your ideal weight. To lose weight while eating macrobiotically, you needn't count calories; merely follow the standard macrobiotic diet, and eat few, if any, snacks and desserts. To gain weight, do the reverse. Once your weight has stabilized, eat the widest possible variety of recommended foods, while still keeping meals simple.

ELEVEN

The Macrobiotic Kitchen

Your success with the macrobiotic diet begins in the kitchen. Preparing nutritionally balanced and tasty macrobiotic food is an exciting endeavor, especially if you plan to involve your spouse or other family members in this new way of eating. This chapter will describe kitchen equipment and how it is used, basic cooking techniques, and menu planning. These suggestions will not only save you time and energy, but also may mean the difference between mediocre and optimal results.

KITCHEN EQUIPMENT

To begin cooking macrobiotic meals, you may need to make an investment in a few kitchen items. You might have them already, but if not, don't try to do without them. By and large, these items are not costly, and they will pay for themselves in countless ways. A stainless steel pressure cooker is the first piece of equipment you will need. (See Figure 11.1.) It is used often in the

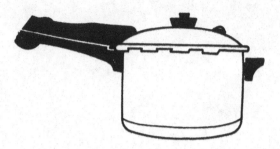

Figure 11.1   Pressure Cooker

macrobiotic kitchen to prepare grains and sometimes beans. The 4-quart size is recommended. In addition, an assortment of stainless steel and cast-iron cooking pots is necessary for cooking soups, vegetables, beans, and grains. Such an assortment might include four stainless-steel saucepans (two 3-quart, one 2-quart, one 1-quart), a 6-quart cast-iron Dutch oven, a cast-iron skillet 9 inches in diameter, and one ovenproof baking dish (3-quart size). For baking, heat-resistant glass or earthenware casseroles, bread pans, and pie plates are best.

You may be accustomed to using aluminum pots and pans, or cookware coated with a nonstick finish. If you use aluminum cookware often, your blood and bones may absorb aluminum, possibly leading to a toxic condition. Metabolic dysfunctions associated with aluminum poisoning include anemia, headaches, liver and kidney problems, and colitis.

The plastic nonstick coating in pots and pans is easily scratched and often flakes off and gets cooked in with food. As the stability of this plastic material in the digestive tract is questionable, and its long-term effects on human health are unknown, it is best to avoid nonstick as well as aluminum cookware.

Metal cooking utensils, especially knives and spoons, are sometimes coated with aluminum, cadmium, lead, or chemical agents during manufacture. Wooden utensils are therefore recommended. Obtain a few inexpensive utensils, such as large wooden spoons or ladles, bamboo rice paddles, a roasting paddle, and chopsticks. (See Figure 11.2.) Stainless steel flatware is

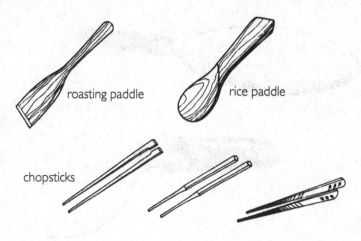

Figure 11.2   Some Recommended Cooking Utensils

appropriate for general table use, but ceramic spoons are especially good for eating soups.

It is best to minimize the use of electric devices in your kitchen. Foods cooked on electric ranges require heavier seasoning, particularly more salt, because they tend to be more bland than foods cooked on a gas range. There is also an increased possibility that foods cooked by electricity will be burned, since it is difficult to control the temperature on electric ranges.

Microwave ovens, in which electromagnetic radiation is used to generate heat, damage the foods cooked in them and can harm the user's health as well. Over a period of years, the consumption of foods cooked on electric ranges or in microwave ovens tends to draw the body out of balance and may lead to health problems. If you replace your electric stove with a gas one, you will notice a difference in your food immediately, and your health will improve as well.

Flat metal flame deflectors with wooden handles are recommended for use when you cook with gas. (See Figure 11.3.) The flame deflector, which is placed under a pot or pressure cooker during slow cooking of grains, helps to distribute the flame more evenly and prevents burning. Metal deflectors are preferable to ones made of asbestos, a known carcinogen.

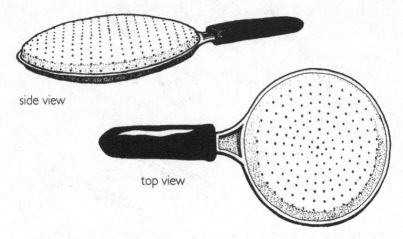

side view

top view

Figure 11.3   Flame Deflector

For preparing vegetables, a natural bristle vegetable scrub brush and a good sharp vegetable knife are indispensable. A Chinese- or Japanese-style knife made of carbon or stainless steel is especially handy for cutting and chopping. In addition, you will need a sharpening stone and some good-quality wooden cutting boards. It is best to use one fairly large board for cutting vegetables and another, smaller one for fish, because wooden boards are somewhat porous and it is difficult to completely remove the fish odors.

To store seeds, grains, beans, and other dried goods, gallon-sized storage containers with covers are excellent. Glass jars and ceramic or wooden containers are best, because unlike plastic or metal, they do not affect the smell or taste of the foods stored in them. Several smaller glass containers with covers for storing teas, condiments, and spices will also be helpful. One more container that you will use often in cooking is a tamari soy sauce dispenser. (See Figure 11.4.)

For washing dried beans, sea vegetables, grains, and seeds before soaking or cooking, you will need a large wire mesh strainer (2- or 3-quart size). This can double as a colander for washing vegetables or draining noodles. A smaller fine mesh strainer is good for washing items such as sesame seeds and millet. It can also be used to strain tea, although a small, inexpensive bam-

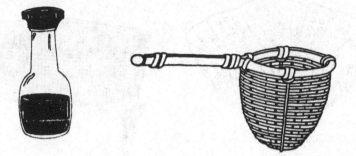

Figure 11.4   Tamari Soy Sauce Dispenser (left)
and Bamboo Tea Strainer

boo tea strainer, used only for teas, is ideal. (See Figure 11.4.) The teas themselves can be brewed in a covered pot or pan—or, of course, in a glass or ceramic teapot.

For grating vegetables and ginger root a handheld grater that permits
fine grating is especially helpful. (See Figure 11.5.) A stainless steel food mill
is convenient for pureeing baby foods and soups. A grinding bowl such as a
Japanese suribachi, with a wooden pestle called a surikogi, is necessary for
making sesame salt and other condiments, sauces, and dressings. (See Figure
11.5.) A 6-inch suribachi is good for regular use.

A steamer basket, a pickle press, and a few inexpensive bamboo mats are
the other kitchen items that are used most regularly in the preparation of

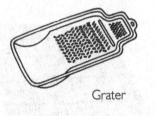

Grater

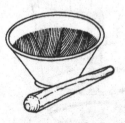

Suribachi and Surikogi

Figure 11.5   Grater (left) and Suribachi with Surikogi

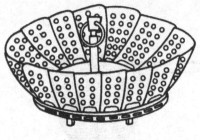

stainless steel steamer

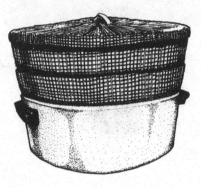

bamboo steamer

Figure 11.6   Steamers

macrobiotic meals. A steamer basket, preferably one made of stainless steel or bamboo, is essential for cooking vegetables and reheating cooked grains. (See Figure 11.6.). A pickle press is useful for preparing pressed salads and pickles; however, you may also make these in a heavy crock, by simply covering the vegetables with a wooden or ceramic plate that fits inside the crock, and setting a weight on top. Bamboo mats will serve you well, especially in the preparation of sushi, a dish made of rice and vegetables or fish rolled in sheets of toasted nori sea vegetable. (See Figure 11.7.)

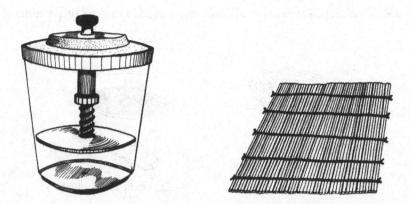

Figure 11.7   Pickle Press (left) and Bamboo Sushi Mat

Of course, you are not limited to using only these kitchen items. But if you use others, make sure they are made of wood, cast iron, stainless steel, glass, or earthenware. If you own a stainless steel wok, it will come in handy for sautéing vegetables and noodles; if not, you may use a stainless steel or cast-iron skillet to serve the same purpose. Electrical appliances such as blenders, popcorn makers, waffle irons, blenders, and juicers are rarely used to make macrobiotic meals.

STOCKING YOUR SHELVES

If you choose to follow the macrobiotic diet, you will be embarking on a whole new way of life. Eventually, you may want to clean out your shelves and cupboards, replacing processed and refined items with whole foods. Almost all of these can be found in a good natural foods store; if they are not available in your area, they can be ordered by mail. Table 11.1 lists the foods and condiments that you may wish to include in your kitchen. If you wish to adopt the macrobiotic way of life more gradually, you may wish to refer to the list of transitional foods in the preceding chapter for suggestions about replacing conventional recipe ingredients with more healthful alternatives.

AT HOME IN YOUR KITCHEN

In macrobiotics, the proper preparation and cooking of food is as important as the food itself. Proper cooking takes into consideration the ever-changing balance of nature: the various seasons and locations in which individual foods grow; their unique flavors, textures, and energetic qualities; and their relationship to the other foods with which they are cooked and eaten. Proper cooking enhances the flavor of foods, stimulates the appetite, and brings the body into balance. Through subtle changes in food variety, cooking techniques, and seasonings, the macrobiotic cook can continually build health

Table 11.1 Foods to Have on Hand

Beans	Adzuki, black beans, black soybeans, chickpeas, kidney beans, lentils, lima beans, pinto beans, soybeans, split peas, whole dried peas
Beverages	Apple juice, bancha tea, grain coffee, mu tea, roasted barley tea, spring water
Condiments and seasonings	Barley malt, brown rice vinegar, gomashio, kelp-sesame salt, miso, nori condiment, raisins and other dried fruits, roasted sea vegetable powders, tamari soy sauce, tekka, umeboshi plums, yinnie (rice) syrup
Dried fruits	Apples, apricots, cherries, currants, peaches, pears, prunes, raisins
Dried or powdered vegetables	Daikon, ginger, onions, parsley, shiitake mushrooms
Flour and flour products	Buckwheat, cornmeal, rye, sourdough bread, tortillas, unyeasted bread, unleavened crackers, whole wheat (regular and pastry)
Grains	Barley, bulghur wheat, corn, couscous, kasha (roasted buckwheat groats), millet, rice cakes, rolled oats, short and medium grain brown rice, sweet brown rice, wheat-berries, whole oats, whole rye
Noodles	Ramen (whole wheat, rice, buckwheat), soba (buckwheat), somen (fine whole wheat), udon (whole-wheat), other whole-wheat pastas
Sea vegetables	Agar-agar, arame, dulse, hijiki, Irish moss, kelp, kombu, nori, wakame, powdered sea vegetables
Seeds and nuts	Pumpkin, sesame, sunflower; almonds, chestnuts, pecans, roasted peanuts, walnuts

Fish and seafoods	A changing variety, including carp, clams, cod, flounder, haddock, halibut, herring, oysters, scallops, scrod, shrimp, smelts, sole, trout, and other salt-water and freshwater white-meat fish
Fruits	A seasonal variety, including apples, apricots, blackberries, blueberries, cantaloupe, cherries, grapes, honeydew melon, peaches, pears, plums, raspberries, strawberries, and watermelon
Oils	Unrefined corn, safflower, sesame (dark and light); peanut butter, sesame butter, tahini
Sweeteners	Apple juice or cider, barley malt, fresh fruit, rice malt, yinnie (rice) syrup
Vegetables	Broccoli, Brussels sprouts, burdock, cabbages, carrots, cauliflower, daikon, daikon greens, kale, leeks, lettuce, lotus root, mushrooms, mustard greens, parsley, parsnips, pumpkins, radishes, rutabagas, scallions, snow peas, squashes, turnip greens, watercress
Miscellaneous	Amasake, dried tofu, fu, ginger, horseradish, mochi, natto, natural mustard, peas, pickled vegetables, popping corn, sauerkraut, seitan, tempeh, tofu

and vitality, while maintaining his or her overall physical and mental balance.

With your kitchen equipment ready and your shelves and refrigerator stocked, you are all set to practice the techniques of macrobiotic food preparation. The ways in which foods are washed, soaked, cut, cooked, and served are all important.

Washing and Soaking

It is important that vegetables be thoroughly washed before they are cut and cooked. It is best not to wash them, however, until you are ready to use them, as they lose their freshness more quickly after they have been washed.

To wash root or ground vegetables, use a natural-bristle vegetable scrubber to remove all soil and dust. Scrub firmly in cold water, being careful not to remove the skin, especially of root vegetables, as it is very nutritious.

It is best to submerge leafy greens in cold water for several seconds before washing them quickly but thoroughly (also with cold water) to remove any sand or soil. Discard any damaged or discolored leaves before washing.

Rinse the sea vegetables wakame, hijiki, arame, and dulse with cold water two or three times. (Instead of rinsing kombu, wipe it with a clean damp cloth.) In most cases, it is also appropriate to soak sea vegetables in cold water for several minutes. Soaking sea vegetables lowers their sodium content, rinses away any dust, and softens them so that they may be sliced easily. Do not soak arame, however, as it will lose much of its flavor and nutritional value.

Before washing grains, place them in a shallow dish or pie plate and remove any stones, sticks, and discolored or damaged grains. To wash grains, place them in a large bowl, cover them with cold water, quickly hand-agitate them, and then pour off the water. Repeat this procedure two or three times, until the water is fairly clear. Then pour the grains into a strainer and give them a final quick rinse under cold water to remove any remaining dust and dirt particles. Dried beans also may be washed in this manner.

Most beans are best soaked for six to eight hours before they are cooked, but it is not necessary to soak lentils and split peas, as they cook very quickly. Soaking is generally recommended because it softens the beans, makes them more digestible, and shortens cooking times. For the same reasons, it may sometimes be appropriate to soak grains such as whole barley, rye, oats, wheat, and (very occasionally) brown rice for six to eight hours.

To soak beans or grains, wash them, place them in a bowl, cover them with water, and set them aside for six to eight hours. Discard the water from soaking beans; the water from soaking grains can be used in cooking to provide additional flavor and nutritive value.

Cutting

Cutting vegetables into various shapes before cooking speeds cooking time (which conserves energy), makes them manageable for eating, and improves texture and appearance. Two other important reasons for cutting vegetables into different shapes are seasonal differences and variety. For instance, if you stir-fry vegetables for a light summer noodle and vegetable dish, you can reduce the amount of time you need to spend in the kitchen by cutting them very thin so that they cook quickly. As for variety, there is no doubt that cutting vegetables into creative shapes adds to their sensory appeal and stimulates the appetite for wholesome fare.

COOKING TECHNIQUES

Macrobiotic cooking differs significantly from several popular cooking styles. In America and parts of Europe, for example, the main ingredient of a meal—usually meat, poultry, or fish—is generally prepared in large pieces, highly seasoned, and served with one or two cooked vegetables, or perhaps with potatoes and a raw salad.

In contrast, the main ingredient of a macrobiotic meal—whole grains—is surrounded by several appealing side dishes made from whole natural ingredients, creating a harmonious combination of flavors, colors, and textures.

Macrobiotic cooking may require more detailed instructions and keener attention to the actual cooking process than you may be accustomed to giving. The simple mixtures and proper cooking methods are important because they take the place of overpowering seasonings and spices in flavoring food. The cooking techniques that are used most regularly in macrobiotic cooking are pressure-cooking, boiling, steaming, nishime (waterless cooking), water-sautéing, pickling, and pressing. Methods that are used less frequently are oil-sautéing, stir-frying, deep frying, baking, and broiling. Raw foods are also used occasionally.

Cooking Whole Grains

To pressure-cook whole grains, wash them and place them in the pressure cooker along with the amount of water specified in the recipe. Add a pinch of sea salt, close the cooker, and bring it up to pressure. Reduce the flame to medium-low and place a metal flame deflector underneath the cooker to keep the grains from burning. Allow the grain to cook for the amount of time specified in the recipe. For basic information about the operation and maintenance of your pressure cooker, read the manufacturer's instructions.

To boil whole grains, wash them and put them in a pot. Add the amount of cold water specified in the recipe and a pinch of sea salt. Cover the pot, bring the water to a boil, and then reduce the flame to low. Place a metal flame deflector underneath the pot to prevent burning. Let the grains cook, undisturbed, for the amount of time specified in the recipe. It is best not to stir whole grains while they are cooking.

After grains are cooked, remove them from the heat and allow them to sit undisturbed in the pot or pressure cooker for four to five minutes. You may wish to cook extra grains to be reheated for lunch the next day. Leftover grains can be stored in the refrigerator for several days.

Steaming is not suggested as a way of cooking whole grains, but it is a good method for reheating leftovers. If you use a stainless-steel steamer basket, simply place the steamer in about half an inch of water in the pot. Add cooked grain, cover the pot, and bring it to a boil. Reduce the flame to low and steam for five minutes or so, until the grain is hot. If you use a bamboo steamer, the same method applies, but you may wish to place the grains on a dinner plate or saucer inside the steamer to prevent them from falling through. If grains are steamed too long, they will get somewhat soggy.

Preparing Quick-Cooking Grains and Whole-Grain Noodles

Precooked grains such as couscous or bulghur wheat are simple to prepare, and they cook quickly. Prepare bulghur wheat by adding it to the amount of boiling water specified in the recipe. Add a pinch of sea salt, cover the pot, and reduce the flame to low. Cook for five to ten minutes, then turn the flame off and let the wheat sit, undisturbed, for about twenty minutes. Remove and fluff up with a spoon. Couscous may be made in the same manner, but the cooking time is less.

The best way to cook whole-grain noodles is quickly, over moderately high heat. Be sure to use plenty of water in a large pot to prevent the noodles from sticking to one another. Bring the water to a boil, add the noodles, and cook them, uncovered, until they are tender. Break a noodle apart and check the center to see if it is cooked through. Drain cooked noodles and rinse them immediately with cold water.

Cooking Beans

Most beans take longer to cook than whole grains. To prepare the smaller beans, such as split peas and lentils, wash them and add them to the amount of cold water specified in the recipe. Cover the pot, bring them to a boil, and reduce the flame to low. Checking occasionally to make sure that the beans have enough water, cook them for the specified amount of time. Uncover the pot, add sea salt, and continue to cook, uncovered, over a low flame, until excess water is boiled off.

Beans such as adzuki beans, kidney beans, pinto beans, chickpeas, and soybeans are best when they are washed and soaked overnight prior to cooking. To prepare them, pour off the water from soaking the beans and place them in a pot. Add the amount of cold water specified in the recipe, along with a strip of kombu sea vegetable. Cover the pot, turn the flame to low, and cook for the specified amount of time, checking occasionally to make sure that the beans have enough water. Uncover the pot, add seasoning such as sea salt, miso, or tamari, and continue to cook over low flame until excess water is boiled off.

Beans take less time when cooked in a pressure cooker. With the exception of split peas, lentils, and black soybeans, all types of beans can generally be pressure-cooked. Place soaked beans, kombu, and water in the pressure cooker, cover, and bring it up to pressure. Reduce the flame to low and cook for the amount of time specified in the recipe. Remove the pressure cooker from heat and allow the pressure to drop before adding seasoning such as sea salt, miso, or tamari. Boil off excess water over a low flame before serving the beans.

Beans are best when cooked until very soft. Undercooked, starchy-tasting beans are hard to digest. Soaking the beans overnight before cooking helps to soften them and removes gas-producing compounds. Cooking the beans with kombu also makes them easier to digest. Leftover beans can be added to soups or fried grains, or reheated in a pan with a little water.

Cooking Vegetables

There are many ways to prepare appealing vegetable dishes, including boiling, steaming, sautéing, nishime (waterless cooking), baking, and tempura (deep-frying).

To boil vegetables, simply place one-half to one inch of water in a pot, bring the water to a boil, and add the vegetables. Cook until the vegetables are moist and tender, then remove them and spread them out in a bowl to cool slightly before serving.

To steam vegetables, wash, cut, and then place them in a steamer basket. You may use either a collapsible stainless-steel steamer that is set down in the pot or a bamboo steamer that rests on top. Place about one-half to one inch of water in the pot and bring the water to a boil. Cover the steamer and steam the vegetables over a medium flame until they become tender.

When using a stainless-steel steamer, make certain that the steamer basket is above the level of the water. Bamboo steamers have separate sections so that you can stack your vegetables, placing the heavier and thicker ones in the bottom layer and then adding the lighter, leafy vegetables to the top layer a short time later. Steamed vegetables are often crisper than boiled ones.

You may wish to save the water left over from steaming or boiling vegetables for use in soups and recipes requiring vegetable stock. Pour the water into an open jar, let it cool, cover it, and refrigerate. The water will keep for several days.

To sauté, lightly brush a cast-iron skillet, wok, or stainless-steel frying pan with sesame oil. For well-done, tender vegetables, heat the skillet, add the vegetables, and cook them over a moderately low flame. Use a high flame if you want crisper, more quickly cooked sautéed vegetables.

To flavor sautéed vegetables and to make the oil easier to digest, you may wish to add a pinch of sea salt at the beginning of cooking or a little tamari soy sauce at the end of cooking. Stir the vegetables occasionally while you are sautéing, and add a little water if necessary to prevent them from sticking.

In most cases, sautéed vegetables are best if they remain crisp, but not raw. In some cases, they may be cooked soft. Generally, greens are best sautéed very quickly, while roots require a little more time. Thicker cuts of root vegetables require more cooking time than thinner ones. Stir-fried vegetables are prepared like sautéed vegetables, except that the flame is turned slightly higher, and they are stirred frequently until done. They should remain fairly crisp.

Another important cooking method is the nishime style, which is also known as waterless cooking. Nishime style is a superb way of cooking vegetables without adding oil or allowing nutrients to escape into boiling or steaming water. This cooking method is often recommended for people with illness.

To prepare nishime, place a couple of strips of soaked and sliced kombu sea vegetable in a pot with a heavy lid. Cut vegetables such as carrots, turnips, daikon, onions, burdock, winter squash, or cabbage into two-inch chunks. Place any combination of these on top of the kombu and add one-half to one inch of water. Add a pinch of sea salt, cover the pot, and place over high flame until the water boils. Reduce flame to low and cook for about twenty-five minutes or until vegetables are tender. Season with a small amount of tamari soy sauce and continue to cook about ten minutes longer or until almost all of the liquid is gone. Mix the vegetables to coat them with any remaining tamari-seasoned juice, remove, and serve.

Other foods that may be included with vegetables in nishime-style cooking are tempeh, fu, dried or fresh tofu, and (as long as you are not cooking for anybody who has a serious illness) pan-fried or deep-fried tofu.

Baking is an especially appropriate method of cooking winter vegetables such as pumpkin or squash. Wash the squash, cut it in half, and place it with the flat side down on a lightly oiled baking sheet. Bake at 375°F until soft. If you are making an oven casserole or vegetable pie, you may steam the vegetables lightly or boil them briefly before baking them in a covered dish.

PLANNING MACROBIOTIC MEALS

The aim of macrobiotic cooking is to achieve balance and harmony in the body and with the environment. When high-quality natural ingredients are properly prepared, in a calm, peaceful, and loving manner, the result is balanced food that will foster a healthy, balanced condition.

Your challenge as a macrobiotic cook will be in preparing and serving dishes that complement one another in a lively unity—not merely in terms of flavor, but nutritionally and visually as well. The well-planned and well-prepared meal will be as pleasing to the eye as it is to the palate. So whether you are arranging a complete meal on each plate or simply placing steamed broccoli in a bowl, try to employ your creative talents. A wide variety of serving dishes and trays will help you to vary the presentation of the food you cook. Of course, it is not necessary (or desirable) to have complicated dishes or arrangements of food every day.

Designing a macrobiotic meal is likely to require a bit more thinking ahead and planning than you are used to. You may find Figure 1.2 in Chapter 1 and the sample menus in Table 11.2 to be helpful guides in planning daily menus.

If you read and follow the recipe directions carefully, your first meal will be as good as the rest. As you become more comfortable in your new kitchen, don't be afraid to improvise, using the macrobiotic ingredients discussed throughout this book. You will soon be preparing meals so delectable that people will think you have been cooking this way all your life.

One of the most important aspects of planning and preparing a macrobiotic meal is timing. In general, whole grains, beans, sea vegetables such as kombu and hijiki, and baked vegetables take the longest to cook, anywhere from fifty minutes to two and a half hours. Pressure-cooking takes less time, but cooking all your food in a pressure cooker to save time isn't a good idea, as using a variety of cooking techniques is important to macrobiotic cooking and to your health. Miso soup and boiled, steamed, and sautéed foods take about ten to fifteen minutes to prepare, as do noodles, couscous, tofu, natto, and tempeh. Nishime takes about thirty to forty minutes. As the recipes in Chapter 12 indicate, foods such as pickles, sourdough breads, pressed salads, and sauerkraut may take anywhere from several hours to a few days to ferment.

Table 11.2 Sample Menus

MENU 1

Breakfast	Lunch	Dinner
Soft rice cereal	Millet croquettes	Lentil soup
Fried tofu	Chinese-style vegetables	Pressure-cooked brown rice
Steamed broccoli	Rice-bran pickles	Kinpura carrots and burdock
Bancha tea	Bancha tea	Boiled mustard greens
		Red radish pickles
		Raisin-nut cookies
		Grain coffee

MENU 2

Breakfast	Lunch	Dinner
Miso soup	Carrot and watercress sushi	French onion soup
Whole oats with raisins	Steamed kale	Pressure-cooked brown rice
Broccoli pickles	Fried tempeh with ginger	with adzuki beans
Gomashio	Bancha tea	Boiled turnip greens
Bancha tea		Nishime vegetables
		Cucumber pickles
		Grain coffee

MENU 3

Breakfast	Lunch	Dinner
Crisp brown-rice cereal	Udon and broth	Pressure-cooked brown rice
Amasake	Boiled tempeh and scallions	and barley
Chinese cabbage pickles	Garden salad	Watercress soup
Grain coffee	Bancha tea	Ginger-broiled scallops
		Boiled salad with tempeh
		Nori condiment
		Blueberry couscous cake
		Bancha tea

MENU 4

Breakfast	Lunch	Dinner
Buckwheat pancakes	Whole-grain and vegetable patties	Pressure-cooked brown rice
Applesauce	Grated daikon	Chickpea soup
Steamed Chinese cabbage	Steamed kale and carrots	Hijiki salad
Onion pickles	Bancha tea	Boiled watercress
Bancha tea		Sautéed burdock with sesame seeds
		Bancha tea

MENU 5

Breakfast	Lunch	Dinner
Soft millet and squash	Fried rice and vegetables	Pressure-cooked brown rice and millet
Toasted nori strips	Daikon pickles	Scrambled tofu
Sauerkraut	Grain coffee	Puréed squash soup
Bancha tea		Boiled broccoli
		Pressed salad
		Stewed pears
		Bancha tea

MENU 6

Breakfast	Lunch	Dinner
Soft barley	Rice balls or triangles	Pressure-cooked brown rice
Miso soup with wakame and daikon	Watercress sushi	seitan-barley soup
Steamed collard greens	Broiled tofu	Watercress salad
Bancha tea	Grain coffee	Dried daikon and kombu
		Cucumber pickles
		Apple-raisin kanten
		Bancha tea

MENU 7		
Breakfast	Lunch	Dinner
Mochi	Fried udon and vegetables	Pressure-cooked brown rice
Grated daikon	Steamed kale	and wheatberries
Toasted nori strips	Grain coffee	Clear broth
Boiled Chinese cabbage		Adzuki beans with kombu
Bancha tea		and squash
		Arame with carrots and
		onions
		Boiled mustard greens
		Boiled red radishes with
		umeboshi-kuzu sauce
		Bancha tea

The sample menus in Table 11.2 are intended as a guide for beginners. You can experiment further and create lively and tasty combinations of your own. If you are committed to the macrobiotic way of cooking, you have a lifetime of learning ahead of you, for the possibilities are limitless. Along this line, cooking classes offered by macrobiotic cooks can be invaluable.

TWELVE

Recipes

The recipes in this chapter will introduce you to the delicious variety of macrobiotic cooking. They are generally appropriate for people in good health who live in a temperate, four-season climate. Many of the basic cooking techniques discussed in Chapter 11, including boiling, steaming, pressure-cooking, sautéing, and nishime, are used, and a number of cutting and serving styles are suggested.

Whole grains, vegetables, and beans (legumes) make up 80 to 90 percent of the macrobiotic diet. Recipes emphasizing these ingredients are presented first in this chapter. They are followed by a number of recipes for soups and supplementary foods. As a whole, these simple, easy-to-prepare recipes have been selected to provide practical guidelines for a balanced and nutritious way of eating.

Once you familiarize yourself with the recipes, you can locate any one of them quickly by using the index starting on page 255. Each recipe will serve three or four people. If you are cooking for more than four people, it will take a little more time to wash, cut, and cook the larger volume of food. Use larger pots, and adjust the recipes as needed. If any food is left over, it can be reheated and served the following day.

Of course, the recipes in this chapter are only a small sampling of the infinite possibilities that you may explore in the world of macrobiotic cooking. When you become adept at basic cooking styles, techniques, and menu planning, you may wish to consult other sources for additional recipes and information about macrobiotic food preparation. There are a number of excellent macrobiotic cookbooks available, and classes with experienced macrobiotic cooking instructors are most helpful.

GRAINS

Grain Entrées

PRESSURE-COOKED BROWN RICE

1 cup brown rice
1¼–1½ cups water
pinch of sea salt

- Wash rice and place in pressure cooker. Add water and cook over low flame for 10–15 minutes. Add sea salt and place cover on pressure cooker. Turn flame to high and bring cooker up to pressure. Reduce flame to medium-low, place flame deflector under cooker, and cook for 50 minutes.
- Remove cooker from flame and allow pressure to come down. Remove cover and let rice sit in cooker for 4–5 minutes. Place rice in a wooden bowl and serve.

Pressure-Cooked Brown Rice with Adzuki Beans

¼ cup adzuki beans
1½–1¾ cups water
1 cup brown rice
pinch of sea salt

· Wash adzuki beans and place in a saucepan with 1½–1¾ cups of water. Bring to a boil, cover, and reduce flame to medium-low. Simmer for 15–20 minutes. Remove from flame and allow beans to cool. Reserve cooking water.
· Wash rice and place in pressure cooker. Add cooled beans and cooking water (make sure there are 1½–1¾ cups left; if necessary, add fresh water to make up the difference).
· Cook over low flame for 15–20 minutes. Add sea salt and place cover on pressure cooker. Turn flame to high and bring cooker up to pressure. Reduce flame to medium-low, place flame deflector under cooker, and cook for 50 minutes.
· Remove from flame and allow pressure to come down. Remove cover and let rice sit in cooker for 4–5 minutes. Place rice in a wooden bowl, and serve.

Pressure-Cooked Brown Rice and Barley

¾ cup brown rice
¼ cup pearled barley
1½ cups water
pinch of sea salt

- Wash rice and barley and place in pressure cooker. Add water. Set aside to soak for 4–5 hours. After soaking grains, cook over low flame for 10–15 minutes. Add sea salt and place cover on pressure cooker. Turn flame to high and bring cooker up to pressure. Reduce flame to medium-low, place flame deflector under cooker, and cook for 50 minutes.
- Remove cooker from flame and allow pressure to come down. Remove cover and let rice and barley sit in cooker for 4–5 minutes. Place grains in a wooden bowl, and serve.

PRESSURE-COOKED BROWN RICE
AND WHEATBERRIES

¼ cup wheatberries
¾ cup brown rice
1½ cups water
pinch of sea salt

- Soak wheatberries in water for 6–8 hours or dry-roast them. Wash rice and place in pressure cooker. Add water. Set aside to soak for 4–5 hours. After soaking wheatberries and rice, cook over low flame for 10–15 minutes. Add sea salt and place cover on pressure cooker. Turn flame to high and bring cooker up to pressure. Reduce flame to medium-low, place flame deflector under cooker, and cook for 50 minutes.
- Remove cooker from flame and allow pressure to come down. Remove cover and let wheatberries and rice sit in cooker for 4–5 minutes. Place in a wooden bowl, and serve.

Pressure-Cooked Brown Rice and Millet

¾ cup brown rice
¼ cup millet
1½ cups water
pinch of sea salt

- Wash rice and millet and place in pressure cooker. Add water and cook over medium-low flame for 10–15 minutes. Add sea salt and place cover on pressure cooker. Turn flame to high and bring cooker up to pressure. Reduce flame to medium-low, place flame deflector under cooker, and cook for 50 minutes.
- Remove cooker from flame and allow pressure to come down. Remove cover and let rice and millet sit in cooker for 4–5 minutes. Place grains in a wooden bowl, and serve.

Rice Balls or Triangles

2 sheets toasted nori (page 175)
4 cups pressure-cooked or boiled brown rice
2 umeboshi plums, halved

- Fold both sheets of toasted nori in half and tear along fold. Then fold each section in half again and tear along fold to make a total of 8 equal-sized pieces. Set aside.
- Wet your hands slightly in a dish of water with a pinch of sea salt dissolved in it. Take 1 cup of rice and form it into a ball or triangle by cupping your hands into a V shape. Pack rice firmly to form a solid ball or

triangle. With your thumb, press a hole into the center of the rice and insert ½ umeboshi plum. Firmly pack rice ball or triangle again to close the hole.

- Wet your hands slightly and cover rice ball or triangle with 2 pieces of nori, 1 piece at a time, so that it sticks. You may have to wet your hands occasionally to keep rice and nori from adhering to them, but if you use too much water, the rice balls will lose some of their flavor and spoil relatively quickly.
- Continue making rice balls or triangles until all rice is used (4 rice balls or triangles). Place on a platter and serve.

SESAME-COATED RICE BALLS OR TRIANGLES

4 cups pressure-cooked or boiled brown rice
2 umeboshi plums, halved
½ cup roasted sesame seeds (page 191)

- Wet your hands very slightly. Take about 1 cup of rice and form it into a ball or triangle by cupping your hands into a V shape. Pack rice firmly to form a solid ball or triangle. With your thumb, press a hole into the center of the rice and insert ½ umeboshi plum. Firmly pack rice ball or triangle again to close the hole. Roll in roasted sesame seeds to coat evenly.
- Repeat this process with the remaining ingredients to make 4 rice balls or triangles. Place on a platter and serve.

CUCUMBER SUSHI

4 sheets toasted nori (page 175)
8 cups pressure-cooked brown rice
1 cucumber, sliced lengthwise into strips ½ inch thick
2 tablespoons shiso leaves

- Place a sheet of toasted nori on a bamboo sushi mat. Evenly spread about 2 cups of cooked brown rice over the nori sheet, leaving 1–2 inches at the top edge and about ¼ inch at the bottom edge uncovered. Press rice down firmly with a slightly damp bamboo rice paddle.
- Place 1–2 cucumber strips across the width of the nori sheet, ½–1 inch from the bottom. Next, place 3–4 shiso leaves in a row parallel to the cucumber strips.
- Use both hands to roll the sushi mat into a cylindrical shape, pressing mat firmly against nori and rice. When nori sheet is completely rolled up, wet the top edge lightly with water and press to seal edges tightly. Before unrolling sushi mat, squeeze gently to remove excess liquid.
- Wet a sharp vegetable knife and slice nori roll in half. Wet knife again and slice each half into 4 equal sections (rounds), approximately 1 inch thick. You may need to wet the knife slightly before making each cut. Repeat the entire process with other sheets of nori.
- Arrange sushi on an attractive platter with cut side facing up, showing rice and cucumber, and serve.

Carrot and Watercress Sushi

2 carrots, quartered lengthwise

16 watercress sprigs

4 sheets toasted nori (page 175)

8 cups pressure-cooked brown rice

4 tablespoons roasted sesame seeds (page 191)

- Place about ½ inch of water in a saucepan and bring to a boil. Drop in carrot strips and simmer until tender. Use a slotted spoon or a pair of cooking chopsticks to remove cooked carrots, leaving the water in the pot. Let carrots drain in a colander. Drop watercress sprigs into cooking water, and boil for about 45 seconds. Remove, drain, and spread out on a plate to cool.
- Place a sheet of toasted nori on a bamboo sushi mat. Evenly spread about 2 cups of cooked brown rice over the nori sheet, leaving 1–2 inches at the top edge and about ¼ inch at the bottom edge uncovered. Press rice down firmly with a slightly damp bamboo rice paddle.
- Place 2 strips of carrot across the width of the nori sheet, about an inch or so from the bottom. Next, place 4 sprigs of watercress in a row alongside carrot strips. Sprinkle about 1 tablespoon of roasted sesame seeds on top of the vegetables.
- Use both hands to roll the sushi mat into a cylindrical shape, pressing mat firmly against nori and rice. When nori sheet is completely rolled up, wet the top edge lightly with water and press to seal edges tightly. Before unrolling sushi mat, squeeze gently to remove excess liquid.
- Wet a sharp vegetable knife and slice nori roll in half. Wet knife again and slice each half into 4 equal sections (rounds), approximately 1 inch thick. You may need to wet the knife slightly before making each cut. Repeat the entire process with other sheets of nori.
- Arrange sushi on an attractive platter with cut side facing up, showing carrot and watercress, and serve.

TEMPEH-SAUERKRAUT SUSHI

1 pound tempeh

water

tamari, to taste

4 sheets toasted nori (page 175)

8 cups pressure-cooked brown rice

8 tablespoons sauerkraut

- Slice tempeh into strips about 6 inches long by ¼ wide by ½ thick. Place in a pot with enough water to almost cover. Cover pot, bring water to a boil, and reduce flame to medium-low. Simmer for 15–20 minutes. Season with tamari and continue cooking, uncovered, until all liquid is gone.
- Place a sheet of toasted nori on a bamboo sushi mat. Evenly spread about 2 cups of cooked brown rice over the nori sheet, leaving 1–2 inches at the top edge and about ¼ inch at the bottom edge uncovered. Press rice down firmly with a slightly damp bamboo rice paddle.
- Place 1–2 strips of tempeh across the width of the nori sheet, about an inch or so from the bottom. Place 2 tablespoons of sauerkraut on top of the tempeh.
- Use both hands to roll the sushi mat into a cylindrical shape, pressing mat firmly against nori and rice. When nori sheet is completely rolled up, wet the top edge lightly with water and press to seal edges tightly. Before unrolling sushi mat, squeeze gently to remove excess liquid.
- Wet a sharp vegetable knife and slice nori roll in half. Wet knife again and slice each half into 4 equal sections (rounds), approximately 1 inch thick. You may need to wet the knife slightly before making each cut. Repeat the entire process with other sheets of nori.
- Arrange sushi on an attractive platter with cut side facing up, and serve.

Mochi

1 cup sweet brown rice
1–1¼ cups water
pinch of sea salt
grated daikon, as garnish
toasted nori strips, as garnish

- Wash sweet rice and place in pressure cooker. Add water. Set aside to soak for 4–6 hours. After soaking sweet rice, add sea salt and place cover on pressure cooker. Turn flame to high and bring cooker up to pressure. Reduce flame to medium-low, place flame deflector under cooker, and cook for 50 minutes.

- Remove cooker from flame and allow pressure to come down. Let sweet rice sit in cooker for 4–5 minutes before placing it in a thick wooden bowl. Pound rice with a heavy wooden pestle until all grains are crushed and rice becomes very sticky. You may need to wet the pestle occasionally, but do not use too much water. Good mochi takes about 1 hour to pound.

- After pounding rice, oil or flour a cookie sheet (use rice flour) and spread rice out to dry for 1–2 days. Store dried mochi in refrigerator or in a cool dry place.

- To toast mochi after it has dried properly, slice into 2-inch squares and place in skillet. Turn flame to medium-low and cover skillet. Toast until mochi is golden brown, then turn it over and toast other side until golden brown. Remove and serve with grated daikon and a few toasted nori strips. Serve each person 2 or 3 slices of mochi.

Fried Rice and Vegetables

dark sesame oil

1 cup diced onions

¼ medium head cabbage, cut into 1-inch chunks (about 1 cup)

1–2 medium carrots, cut into matchsticks (about ½ cup)

4 cups pressure-cooked brown rice

1–2 tablespoons water

tamari, to taste

1 tablespoon chopped parsley

- Heat a small amount of dark sesame oil in a skillet. Sauté onions over high flame for 3–4 minutes. Reduce flame to medium-low and layer cabbage, carrots, and rice on top. Add 1–2 tablespoons water.
- Cover skillet, reduce flame to low, and cook until all vegetables are tender and rice is warm and soft. Just before vegetables are done, season with a little tamari and add chopped parsley. Mix rice with vegetables and continue to cook for another 3–5 minutes.

Udon and Broth

10 cups water (approximately)

1 package (8 ounces) whole-wheat udon noodles

1 kombu strip, 3–4 inches long, soaked

2–3 shiitake mushrooms, soaked, stems removed, and sliced

4 cups water, including water from soaking kombu and shiitake

2–3 tablespoons tamari

4 teaspoons sliced scallions, as garnish

- Place water in a pot and bring to a boil. Stir in udon and cook until noodles are tender and the same color inside and out. Remove udon from heat and place in strainer. Rinse under cold water and allow to drain.
- Place kombu, shiitake, and 4 cups of water in a saucepan. Bring to a boil. Reduce flame to medium-low, cover, and simmer for 5–10 minutes. Remove kombu and set aside for future use. Season soup stock with tamari, reduce flame to low, and simmer for about 5 minutes.
- Place a serving of cooked udon in each individual's bowl and pour about 1 cup of hot broth over udon. Garnish each serving with a teaspoon of sliced scallions, and serve.

FRIED UDON AND VEGETABLES

10 cups water (approximately)
1 package (8 ounces) whole-wheat udon noodles
dark sesame oil
1 medium onion, cut into half-moons
1 celery stalk, sliced diagonally
1 carrot, cut into matchsticks
tamari, to taste

- Place about 10 cups of water in a pot and bring to a boil. Stir in udon and cook until noodles are tender and the same color inside and out. Remove udon from heat and place in strainer. Rinse under cold water and allow to drain.
- Heat a small amount of dark sesame oil in a skillet. Add onion and sauté for 2–3 minutes over fairly high flame, stirring to cook evenly and prevent burning. Add celery and carrot and sauté for 3–4 minutes. Place noodles on top of vegetables, and cover skillet. Reduce flame to low and cook until vegetables are tender.
- Remove cover and season with a little tamari. Mix and sauté for 3–4 minutes longer. Remove, place in a serving bowl, and serve.

MILLET CROQUETTES

4 cups pressure-cooked millet
1 medium onion, diced (about 1 cup)
sesame oil
1 recipe Chinese Style Vegetables (page 152)

- In a bowl, mix millet and diced onion thoroughly. Wet your hands slightly with cold water. Take about ½ cup of millet mixture and press firmly into a ball. Make sure that ball is packed firmly, or it will fall apart while frying.
- Place 2–3 inches of sesame oil in a pot and turn flame to medium. Do not allow oil to smoke or boil. Test temperature by dropping a small amount of millet into it. If oil is not hot enough, millet will stay at the bottom of the pot. If oil is too hot, millet will sink to the bottom but rise back to the surface immediately. If oil is at just the right temperature, millet will first sink to the bottom and then rise to the surface in a few seconds. When oil is at the right temperature, place 2–3 millet balls in pot and deep-fry until golden brown. Remove croquettes and drain.
- Continue to form balls and deep-fry them until all millet is used (8 croquettes). Place 2 croquettes in each individual's bowl. Pour the sauce from Chinese-Style Vegetables recipe over them. Garnish with scallions, if desired, and serve.

HOMEMADE SEITAN

3½ pounds whole-wheat flour (from hard spring or hard winter wheat)

18–20 cups warm spring water

1 kombu strip, 12 inches long, soaked

3–5 tablespoons tamari

- Place flour in a large bowl and add 8–9 cups of warm water to obtain a consistency like oatmeal or cookie batter. Knead for 3–5 minutes, until flour is mixed thoroughly with water. Cover with 4–5 cups of warm water and allow dough to sit for a minimum of 5–10 minutes. Knead again in soaking water for 1 minute. Pour cloudy water into a jar. (This cloudy water is "seitan starch water" and may be saved for use in other recipes.)
- Transfer dough to a large strainer and put the strainer in a large bowl or pot. Pour cold water over the dough and knead in the strainer. Drain off cold water. Pour hot water over the dough and knead again. Alternate between cold and hot water when rinsing and kneading, repeating until bran and gluten are completely separated.
- Gluten should form a sticky mass. Separate it into 5 or 6 pieces and form balls. Drop balls into 6 cups of boiling water and boil for 5 minutes, or until balls rise to the surface. Add kombu and tamari and cook for 35–45 minutes. (The liquid in the pot is "seitan-tamari water" and may be saved for use in other recipes.)
- Slice or cube seitan as called for in a recipe, or store seitan balls in a glass jar in the refrigerator. When stored in the tamari-water mixture, seitan will keep for 4–5 days. The stronger the concentration of tamari, the longer it will keep. Seitan stored in full-strength tamari will keep for several weeks, but it must be soaked in water for about 30 minutes prior to use to remove excess salt.

WHOLE GRAIN AND VEGETABLE PATTIES

4 cups pressure-cooked or boiled millet
1 cup diced onions
½ cup diced carrots
¼ cup diced celery
½ cup cooked seitan diced (page 143)
1 cup water
tamari, to taste
whole-wheat pastry flour or whole-wheat flour (optional)
dark sesame oil
fresh parsley sprigs, as garnish

- In a bowl, mix millet and vegetables thoroughly. Mix in seitan. Add water and a small amount of tamari and mix again. Grain should be moist enough so that you will be able to make patties; if necessary, add a little more water. If grain is too moist, add a little whole-wheat pastry flour until you obtain the right consistency.
- Take 1 handful of grain and vegetable mixture and shape into a patty. Repeat until all grain is gone.
- Heat a moderate amount of sesame oil in a skillet. Place several patties in skillet, cover, and reduce flame to medium-low. Cook until golden brown. Turn patties over and cook until golden brown. Remove and place on a serving platter. Garnish with sprigs of fresh parsley.

Cereals, Pancakes, and Bread

OATMEAL WITH RAISINS

2 cups rolled oats
½ cup raisins
3 cups water
2 pinches of sea salt

- Heat a stainless-steel skillet. Add dry oats, reduce flame to low, and roast oats slowly until they release a nutty fragrance. Stir constantly to avoid burning oats and to roast them evenly.
- Place roasted oats in a pot; add raisins, water, and sea salt. Cover and bring to a boil. Reduce flame to medium-low, place flame deflector under pot, and simmer for 25–30 minutes.
- This cereal may be topped with yinnie (rice) syrup, barley malt, or amasake, or garnished with roasted seeds or nuts.

SOFT RICE CEREAL

1 cup brown rice
5 cups water
pinch of sea salt or ½ umeboshi plum
sliced scallions, as garnish
toasted nori, as garnish

- Wash rice and place in pressure cooker. Add water and sea salt or umeboshi plum. Place cover on pressure cooker and turn flame to high.

Bring cooker up to pressure, place flame deflector underneath, and reduce flame to medium-low. Cook for approximately 50 minutes.

· Remove cooker from flame and allow pressure to come down. Remove cover and place cereal in individual bowls. Garnish with a few sliced scallions and toasted nori strips or squares, and serve.

WHOLE OATS WITH RAISINS

5 cups water
1 cup whole oats
½ cup raisins
pinch of sea salt
gomashio or dulse flakes, as garnish

· Place all ingredients in a pot and bring water to a boil. Cover and reduce flame to very low. Place flame deflector under pot and allow to cook overnight so that cereal becomes very soft and creamy. If you do not want to cook overnight, you may pressure-cook this cereal: place all ingredients in pressure cooker and cook for 50–60 minutes over medium-low flame, as you would for Soft Rice Cereal. Garnish with gomashio (page 182) or dulse flakes.

CRISP BROWN RICE CEREAL

crisp brown rice cereal
amasake

· This prepackaged cereal is available at most natural foods stores. Pour amasake (rice milk) over each individual serving.

Soft Millet and Squash

1 cup millet

5 cups water

1 cup buttercup squash *or* Hokkaido pumpkin, cut into 1-inch
   chunks

pinch of sea salt

chopped scallions or parsley, as garnish (optional)

- Wash millet and place in a dry stainless-steel skillet. Turn flame to low
  and dry-roast millet until it releases a nutty fragrance. Stir constantly to
  roast evenly and prevent burning. Place all ingredients in pressure cooker.
  Cover cooker and bring up to pressure. Place flame deflector under cooker
  and reduce flame to medium-low. Cook for 20 minutes.
- Remove cooker from flame and allow pressure to come down. Serve millet garnished with chopped scallions or parsley, if desired.

Soft Barley

1 cup barley, soaked 6–8 hours
5 cups water
1 kombu strip, 6 inches long, soaked and cut into 1-inch squares
¼ cup chopped scallions
1 sheet toasted nori (page 175), cut into 1-inch squares
pinch of sea salt
tamari, to taste (optional)
chopped scallions, as garnish (optional)
toasted nori, as garnish (optional)
sea salt, as garnish (optional)
2–3 drops tamari, as garnish (optional)

- Place barley, water, and kombu in pressure cooker. Turn flame to high and bring cooker up to pressure. Place flame deflector under cooker and reduce flame to medium-low. Cook for 50 minutes.
- Remove cooker from flame and allow pressure to come down. Place cereal in individual serving dishes and garnish with a few chopped scallions, several squares of toasted nori, sea salt, and 2–3 drops of tamari, if desired. Serve.

Buckwheat Pancakes

1 cup buckwheat flour
½ cup whole-wheat flour or whole-wheat pastry flour
⅛ teaspoon sea salt
1⅓ cups water or apple juice
light sesame oil

- Combine dry ingredients. Add water or apple juice to create the desired consistency for pancakes. Mix very well with a spoon or whisk. Let batter sit in a warm place overnight so that it begins to ferment. This will help the pancakes to rise and become lighter.
- Lightly oil a skillet or pancake griddle with light sesame oil, and heat. Place a small amount of batter on griddle to form a round cake. Fry over medium flame until little air bubbles start to appear on the uncooked side of the pancake. Turn pancake over and fry until golden brown. If flame is too high, pancakes will burn.

SOURDOUGH BREAD

1 cup whole-wheat flour
spring water
8 cups whole-wheat flour *or* 5 cups whole-wheat flour and 3 cups rye flour
¼–½ teaspoon sea salt
2 tablespoons sesame oil (optional)

- Make sourdough starter by adding enough water to 1 cup whole-wheat flour to make a thick batter. Cover with a damp cloth and allow to ferment for 3–4 days in a warm place.
- In a large bowl, mix the rest of the flour and salt together, add oil (if desired), and combine thoroughly by hand. Mix in 1–1½ cups of sourdough starter. Knead 300–350 times. (For variety, you may knead in 1½–2 cups diced onion, 1½–2 cups raisins, or ½–1 cup roasted seeds or nuts.)
- Oil 2 bread pans with sesame oil and dust with flour. Place dough in pans and cover with a damp cloth. Let sit for 8–12 hours in a warm place. After dough has risen, bake at 200°F for 30 minutes and then for 1 hour or so at 350°F.
- Slice and serve.

VEGETABLE DISHES AND SALADS

Vegetable Entrées

BOILED MUSTARD GREENS

½–⅔ pound mustard greens, cut diagonally into 2-inch pieces
(about 4 cups)
water

• Place about 1 inch of water in a pot and bring to a boil. Add mustard greens, cover, and reduce flame to medium-low. Cook for 2–3 minutes so that the greens are slightly crisp and bright green in color. Remove, drain, and place in a serving bowl. You may toss the greens several times with cooking chopsticks or wooden spoons to cool them slightly so that they retain their bright color.
• Mustard greens may also be cooked whole. Cook as described above, remove, drain, and allow to cool slightly. Using both hands, shape greens into a roll or cylindrical shape, and squeeze out most of the liquid. Slice roll into 1½–2-inch pieces and arrange attractively on a serving platter.

BOILED TURNIP GREENS

½–⅔ pound turnip greens, sliced diagonally into 2-inch pieces (about
4 cups)
water
¼ cup roasted sesame or sunflower seeds (page 191) as garnish

- Place about 1 inch of water in a pot and bring to a boil. Add turnip greens, cover, and reduce flame to medium-low. Simmer for 2–3 minutes, until greens are tender but still bright green. Remove, drain, and place in a serving bowl. You may toss the greens several times with wooden spoons or cooking chopsticks to allow them to cool. Sprinkle roasted sesame seeds or sunflower seeds on top for garnish, and serve.

BOILED WATERCRESS

water
2 bunches of watercress
½ lemon, cut into thin half-moons, as garnish

- Place about 1 inch of water in a pot and bring to a boil. Place 1 bunch of watercress in the boiling water. Simmer for 45–50 seconds, stirring or mixing to cook evenly. Use a slotted spoon or a pair of cooking chopsticks to remove cooked watercress, leaving the water in the pot. Drain watercress in a colander. Boil the remaining watercress the same way; remove and drain.
- Place both bunches of watercress on a serving dish or in a bowl. Garnish with lemon slices, either in the center or off to one side.

BOILED BROCCOLI

water
4 cups broccoli florets

- Place about ½ inch of water in a pot and bring to a boil. Add broccoli, cover, and reduce flame to medium-low. Simmer for 2–3 minutes or until broccoli is tender but still bright green and slightly crisp. Remove, drain, and place in a serving bowl.

BOILED CHINESE CABBAGE

4 cups sliced Chinese cabbage, cut diagonally into pieces about 1
  inch wide
water
1 umeboshi plum

- Place about 1 inch of water in a pot and add umeboshi plum. Bring to a
  boil. Add Chinese cabbage, cover, and reduce flame to medium-low.
  Simmer for 1–2 minutes so that cabbage remains crisp. Remove, drain,
  and place in a serving bowl. The umeboshi plum may be saved for use in
  other recipes.

CHINESE-STYLE VEGETABLES

3 cups water
½ medium onion, cut into half-moons (about ½ cup)
3 shiitake mushrooms, soaked, stems removed, and sliced
1–2 medium cup carrots, cut into matchsticks (about ½ cup)
1 cup broccoli florets
1 cup sliced Chinese cabbage, cut diagonally into pieces about 1 inch
  wide
1½ tablespoons kuzu
tamari, to taste

- Place water in a pot and bring to a boil. Add onions and shiitake and reduce flame to medium-low. Cover and simmer for 4–5 minutes. Add
  carrots and broccoli and simmer, covered, for 2–3 minutes. Add Chinese
  cabbage and simmer, covered, for 1 minute more.

- To make sauce, dilute kuzu in 2–3 tablespoons of water. Reduce flame to low and add diluted kuzu, stirring constantly to prevent lumping. When kuzu becomes translucent and creamy, season vegetables with a little tamari to obtain a mild salt taste. Serve over croquettes, noodles, or plain rice, or as a vegetable side dish.

BOILED RED RADISHES WITH UMEBOSHI-KUZU SAUCE

2 cups water
4 shiso leaves
1 umeboshi plum
2 cups trimmed red radishes
3 tablespoons kuzu
1 tablespoon sliced scallions or parsley, as garnish

- Place water, shiso leaves, umeboshi plum, and radishes in a pot and bring water to a boil. Cover, reduce flame to medium-low, and simmer until radishes are tender. Remove and drain radishes and shiso leaves, reserving cooking water. Set umeboshi plum aside. Place radishes in a shallow serving bowl. Chop shiso leaves and set aside.
- Dilute kuzu in a few tablespoons of water and pour into cooking water. The water should be light red. Stir constantly to avoid lumping. When sauce becomes thick and creamy, remove from flame and pour over radishes. Place chopped shiso leaves in the center of the radishes. Sprinkle scallions or parsley on top for garnish, and serve.

Quickly Boiled Watercress and Carrots

water

1 carrot, thinly sliced on a diagonal

2 bunches watercress

- Place 1 inch of water in a pot and bring to a boil. Cook carrots for 50–60 seconds. Use a slotted spoon to remove carrots, leaving the water in the pot. Drain carrots in a colander. Simmer watercress for 50 seconds, stirring or mixing quickly to cook evenly. Remove watercress, drain, and place on cutting board. Slice into 2-inch pieces. Mix carrots and watercress in a serving bowl. Serve with Umeboshi-Sesame Dressing (page 185).

Watercress Sushi

water

4 bunches of watercress

4 sheets toasted nori (page 175)

8–12 shiso leaves

½ cup roasted sesame or sunflower seeds (page 191)

- Place about 1 inch of water in a pot and bring to a boil. Boil watercress for about 50 seconds, stirring or mixing to cook evenly. Remove watercress, drain it, and rinse it under cold water to stop the cooking process and keep the bright green color. Using both hands, squeeze out excess water; set watercress on a plate.
- Place a sheet of toasted nori on a bamboo sushi mat. Take 1 bunch of watercress and spread it evenly over the nori sheet. Cover about ¾ of

the sheet, leaving 2 inches at the top edge and 1 inch at the bottom edge uncovered.

- Place 2–3 shiso leaves in a straight line across the watercress. Sprinkle about ⅛ cup of the sesame or sunflower seeds in a straight line on top of the shiso leaves.
- Use both hands to roll the sushi mat into a cylindrical shape, pressing mat firmly against nori and rice. When nori sheet is completely rolled up, wet the top edge lightly with water and press to seal edges tightly. Before unrolling sushi mat, squeeze gently to remove excess liquid.
- Wet a sharp vegetable knife and slice nori roll in half. Wet knife again and slice each half into 4 equal sections (rounds), approximately 1 inch thick. You may need to wet the knife slightly before making each cut. Repeat the entire process with other sheets of nori.
- Arrange sushi on an attractive platter with cut side facing up, and serve.

STEAMED BROCCOLI

water
4 cups broccoli florets

- Place about 1 inch of water in a pot. Set a steamer down inside the pot. Place broccoli in steamer, cover pot, and bring to a boil. Reduce flame to medium-low and steam broccoli several minutes, until it is tender but still firm and bright green. Remove and place in a serving bowl.

Steamed Kale

water

⅔ pound kale, sliced diagonally (about 4 cups)

tamari, to taste (optional)

- Place about 1 inch of water in a pot. Set a steamer down inside the pot and bring water to a boil. Place kale in steamer. Cover, reduce flame to medium-low, and steam for 1–2 minutes. Sprinkle several drops of tamari (if desired) on the kale and mix. Cover and steam for another minute or so, until kale is tender but slightly crisp and bright green. Remove and place in a serving dish.

Steamed Chinese Cabbage

water

4 cups sliced Chinese cabbage, cut into pieces 1–1½ inches wide

- Place about 1 inch of water in a pot. Set a steamer down inside the pot and bring water to a boil. Add Chinese cabbage. Cover and steam for 2 minutes, so that cabbage is slightly crisp. Remove and place in a serving bowl.

Steamed Kale and Carrots

water

2–3 medium carrots, thinly sliced on a diagonal (about 1 cup)

½ pound kale, stems and greens, sliced diagonally (about 3 cups)

¼ cup roasted sunflower seeds (page 191)

- Place about 2 inches of water in a pot. Set a bamboo steamer on top of the pot and bring water to a boil. Place carrots in steamer, cover, and steam for 3–4 minutes. Remove carrots and place in a serving bowl.
- Make sure that the kale stems are sliced thinner than the leaves, so that they will cook evenly. Place stems in steamer, cover, and steam for 1 minute. Add kale greens and steam for 2–3 minutes. Remove steamed kale and mix in with carrots. Mix in roasted sunflower seeds, and serve.

Steamed Collard Greens

water

½ onion, cut into thin half-moons (about ½ cup)

½ pound collard greens, thinly sliced on a diagonal (about 3 cups)

- Place about 1 inch of water in a pot. Set a steamer down inside the pot and bring water to a boil. Add onions and collard greens. Cover and reduce flame to medium-low. Steam for 2–3 minutes, until collards are tender and bright green. Remove and place in a serving bowl.

KINPURA CARROTS AND BURDOCK

dark sesame oil
1 cup sliced burdock, cut into matchsticks or shaved
5–6 medium carrots, cut into matchsticks (about 2 cups)
water
tamari, to taste

- Heat a small amount of dark sesame oil in a cast-iron or stainless-steel skillet. Sauté burdock over fairly high flame for 3–4 minutes. Place carrots on top of burdock, add several drops of water, and cover skillet. Reduce flame to medium-low. Simmer several minutes, until carrots and burdock are tender. Season with a little tamari and simmer 2–3 minutes longer. Remove cover and cook off any remaining liquid. Mix carrots and burdock, remove from flame, and place in a serving bowl.

SAUTÉED BURDOCK WITH SESAME SEEDS

dark sesame oil
3 cups sliced burdock, cut into matchsticks or shaved
water
½ cup sesame seeds
brown rice vinegar
tamari, to taste

- Heat a small amount of dark sesame oil in a skillet. Place burdock in skillet and sauté over fairly high flame for 4–5 minutes. Add a few drops of water to lightly cover the bottom of the skillet. Cover and reduce flame to medium-low. Cook until burdock is tender. Remove cover and cook off any remaining liquid.

- Dry-roast sesame seeds in a stainless steel skillet, until they are golden brown and release a nutty fragrance. Stir seeds back and forth constantly to keep them from burning. Place roasted seeds in a suribachi, and grind until they are about half crushed.

- Mix in a few drops of brown rice vinegar and several drops of tamari. Add enough water to make a thick paste, and mix. Place burdock in with sesame seeds and mix to thoroughly coat burdock. Remove and place in a serving bowl.

DRIED DAIKON AND KOMBU

dark sesame oil
4 shiitake mushrooms, soaked, stems removed, and sliced
2 kombu strips, 6 inches long, soaked and thinly sliced
2 cups sliced dried daikon, rinsed and soaked
water (include daikon and shittake soaking water)
tamari, to taste

- Heat a small amount of dark sesame oil in a skillet. Add mushrooms and sauté for 3–4 minutes. Add kombu, set daikon on top of kombu, and add enough water to half cover the daikon. Cover skillet and bring water to a boil. Reduce flame to medium-low and simmer for 25–30 minutes. Season with a little tamari to obtain a mild salt taste and continue to cook several minutes longer, until all liquid has evaporated. Mix vegetables and place in a serving bowl.

Nishime Vegetables

1 kombu strip, 6 inches long, soaked and cut into 1-inch squares
1 piece daikon, 4–5 inches long, halved lengthwise and cut into half-moons 1 inch thick
1 cup cubed butternut *or* buttercup squash, cut in 1½-inch chunks
1 cup carrot chunks
pinch of sea salt
water
tamari, to taste

• Place kombu in a heavy pot. Place daikon on top of kombu. Set squash on top of daikon, and place carrots on top of squash. Add a pinch of sea salt and about ½ inch of water. Cover pot and bring water to a boil. Reduce flame to low and simmer until vegetables are tender. Add a small amount of tamari and continue to simmer until vegetables are soft and all liquid has evaporated. Mix vegetables with kombu, remove, and place in a serving bowl.

Grated Daikon

1 piece daikon, 6–8 inches long
tamari, to taste
1 fresh parsley sprig or small daikon leaf

• Grate daikon on a flat grater and place in a small serving dish. Place 3 or 4 drops of tamari in the center of the daikon and garnish with a small sprig of fresh parsley or with a small daikon leaf to one side of the dish. Serve each person 1 or 2 tablespoons.

Pickled Vegetables

RED RADISH PICKLES

10–12 red radishes, trimmed
¾ cup water
¼ cup umeboshi vinegar

- Slice radishes into very thin rounds and place in a pickle press. Add water and umeboshi vinegar. Place top on pickle press and screw down. Let sit for at least 2–3 hours.
- You may leave radishes in pickle press for as long as 1–2 days; the longer you leave them, the saltier and stronger-tasting they become. If pickles become too salty, simply rinse with cold water before eating. If pickles are very salty, serve 2–3 slices to each person. If pickles are mild, several pieces are fine. These pickles will keep for about 1 week in the refrigerator or in a cool place.

RICE BRAN PICKLES

4 cups rice bran (nuka)
1 tablespoons sea salt
water
1 piece daikon, 12–14 inches long, quartered lengthwise

- Place rice bran in a dry skillet. Stirring constantly to prevent burning, roast for several minutes over low flame until a nutty fragrance is released. Remove from flame and allow to cool. When rice bran is cool, place it in a large ceramic or wooden crock or keg. Mix in sea salt and add enough cold water to form a very thick, slightly dry paste. Cut each piece of daikon in half, to obtain a total of 8 pieces, and place them in the keg, making sure that they are completely covered with rice bran paste. Cover the top of the crock or keg with clean cotton cheesecloth to keep dust out.

· Let sit for 5–7 days in a fairly cool place. Mix ingredients daily to pickle evenly and prevent souring. After 5–7 days, remove pickles, rinse under cold water, and slice paper-thin. Arrange on a small serving dish or in a small bowl. Serve 2–3 slices to each person.

BROCCOLI PICKLES

2 cups small broccoli florets
¾ cup water
¼ cup tamari
2 slices fresh ginger

· Place all ingredients in a pickle press or jar. Apply just enough pressure to hold the broccoli under the tamari-water solution. If you use a jar, take a smaller jar or a drinking cup that fits inside and press the pickles by setting a weight in that cup. Let sit for 2–3 days. If pickles are too salty, rinse with cold water before eating. These pickles will keep for about 1 week in a cool place.

QUICK CUCUMBER PICKLES

2 small cucumbers, thinly sliced on the diagonal (about 2 cups)
2 tablespoons brown rice vinegar
½ teaspoon sea salt

- Place all ingredients in a pickle press and mix thoroughly. Place top on pickle press and screw down. When water level rises to pressure plate, release pressure slightly and let sit for 2–3 hours. Remove, squeeze out excess liquid, and place pickles on a serving dish.

CHINESE CABBAGE PICKLES

1 head Chinese cabbage
¼ cup sea salt (approximately)
1 kombu strip (optional)

- Rinse cabbage leaves individually by removing them from the head. Place them in a colander to allow water to drain. When all water has drained off, the cabbage leaves are ready to use.
- Sprinkle a thin layer of sea salt in the bottom of a ceramic crock or wooden keg. If desired, place a strip of kombu at the bottom of the crock, as well. The kombu absorbs water, adds minerals, and changes the taste of the pickles.
- Place a layer of cabbage leaves over the first layer of salt aligned in one direction. Add a thin layer of salt (several pinches are sufficient), and align a layer of leaves in the opposite direction. Repeat layering until all cabbage is used. Finish with a layer of salt.
- Place a plate on top of the last layer of salt. Set several clean, heavy rocks on the plate to press the leaves down.
- If water does not start to come out of the cabbage within 10–12 hours, more salt is needed. When water rises up to the level of the plate, remove some of the weight so that the level drops just below the plate. Check the water level every day and make sure that all is going well.
- Pickles may be eaten after 3–4 days, or they may be left several days longer for a more sour taste. Rinse and slice before serving. Excess salt

can be washed off by dipping pickles in warm water or soaking them for a short time. Store in a cool, dark place.

- If the pickles begin to spoil at any point during the pickling process, add more salt or more pressure, and skim off the mold. It may be necessary to start again with fresh cabbage.

ONION PICKLES

1 medium onion, cut into thin half-moons (about 2 cups)
1 cup water
½ cup tamari

- Place all ingredients in a pickle press. Place top on pickle press and apply just enough pressure to hold onions under the tamari-water solution. Leave pickles for 1–2 days; the longer they sit, the saltier they will become. If they become too salty, rinse under cold water before eating. These pickles will keep for about 1 week in a cool place.

SAUERKRAUT

5 pounds cabbage
⅓ cup sea salt

- Wash and finely shred cabbage. Place it in a wooden keg or ceramic crock and mix sea salt in very well. Place several clean rocks on top of a plate to press the cabbage. Cover with a piece of clean cheesecloth to keep dust out. Within 10 hours, the water level in the keg will rise up to or above the plate. If the level is above the plate, remove some of the weight to make the water recede. Keep sauerkraut in a cool, dark place for 1½–2 weeks. Check it every day to make sure all is going well. If mold begins to form on top, remove and discard it immediately.

- When sauerkraut is ready, rinse it with cold water and place in a serving dish.

DAIKON PICKLES

1½ pounds daikon, cut into thin half-moons (about 2 cups)
1 teaspoon lemon peel matchsticks
¼ teaspoon sea salt

- Place all ingredients in a pickle press and mix thoroughly. Place top on pickle press and screw down. Leave for 2–3 hours. Remove lemon peels and discard. Place the top back on, apply enough pressure to keep the water level just below the pressure plate, and let pickles sit for 1 day. Remove and place in a serving dish.

CUCUMBER PICKLES

10 cups water
⅓ cup sea salt
12–15 cucumbers, quartered lengthwise (about 3 pounds)
2 fresh dill sprigs

- Place water and salt in a large crock or clean glass jar. Stir until salt dissolves. Add cucumbers and dill. Place clean cotton cheesecloth over the top of the crock or jar to allow air in and to keep dust out. Leave in a cool place for 2–3 days. Refrigerate and let sit for 2–3 more days. Place on an attractive serving tray, and serve.
- See also Pressed Salad, page 168.

Salads

Boiled Salad

water

½ onion, cut into thick half-moons

¼ pound kale, sliced into pieces about 1½ inches wide (about 1 cup)

1–2 medium carrots, cut into thin half-moons (about ½ cup)

¼ medium cabbage, cut into 1-inch chunks (about 1 cup)

- Place about 1 inch of water in a pot and bring to a boil. Add the onions and boil for about 1 minute. Use a slotted spoon or a pair of cooking chopsticks to remove onions, leaving the cooking water in the pot. Drain onions in a colander before placing in a large serving bowl. Boil kale in the same water for 1–2 minutes; remove and drain. Place in bowl with onions.

- Then boil carrots in the same water for 1–2 minutes. Remove cooked carrots, drain, and mix in with kale and onions. Finally, cook the cabbage in the boiling water for about 2 minutes. Remove, drain, and mix in with other vegetables. Serve plain or with dressing.

BOILED SALAD WITH TEMPEH

dark sesame oil

1 cup cubed tempeh, cut into 1-inch pieces

2 slices of fresh ginger

water

tamari, to taste

1–2 medium carrots, thinly sliced on a diagonal (about ½ cup)

2 cups broccoli florets

¼ medium cabbage, cut into 1-inch chunks (about 1 cup)

- Heat a small amount of dark sesame oil in a skillet. Place tempeh and ginger in a skillet and sauté for 3–4 minutes over fairly high flame. Add just enough water to cover the bottom of the skillet. Cover skillet and reduce flame to low. Simmer for 25–30 minutes.

- Season with a little tamari for a mild salt taste and continue to cook for 5–10 more minutes. Remove cover and cook off all remaining liquid. Place tempeh in a serving bowl and set ginger aside for use in other dishes.

- Place 1 inch of water in a pot and bring to a boil. Add carrots. Cover and reduce flame to medium-low. Cook for 1–2 minutes. Use a slotted spoon to remove carrots, leaving the cooking water in the pot. Drain carrots in a colander before placing in serving bowl with tempeh. Cook broccoli in the same boiling water for 2–3 minutes, until tender, bright green, and slightly crisp. Remove broccoli, drain, and place in a bowl with carrots and tempeh. Cook cabbage in the boiling water for 2–3 minutes. Remove, drain, and place in bowl with other ingredients. Mix and serve.

Watercress Salad

water

1 cup carrots, cut into matchsticks

3 bunches watercress

- Place 1 inch of water in a pot and bring to a boil. Simmer carrots for 1 minute. Use a slotted spoon to remove carrots, leaving the cooking water in the pot. Drain carrots in a colander before placing in a serving bowl. Cook watercress in the same boiling water for 50 seconds, stirring or mixing to cook evenly. Remove and drain. Toss to cool, or spread apart on a plate. Slice watercress into 2-inch slices and mix in with carrots. Serve with Umeboshi-Scallion Dressing (page 184).

Pressed Salad

2 cups very thinly sliced Chinese cabbage

1 cup sliced cucumbers

½ cup thinly sliced red radishes

¼–⅓ medium onion, cut into very thin half-moons (about ¼ cup)

3 tablespoons brown rice vinegar

½ teaspoon sea salt

- Place all ingredients in a pickle press and mix thoroughly to coat vegetables evenly with vinegar and salt. Place top on pickle press and screw down firmly. The salt causes the water in the vegetables to come out. When water level rises to the pressure plate, release pressure slightly to allow vegetables to absorb salt and vinegar. Let sit for 1–2 hours. Remove vegetables, squeeze out excess liquid, and place in a serving bowl.

GARDEN SALAD

3 cups fresh iceberg or romaine lettuce, sliced or pulled apart
½ cup shredded or coarsely grated carrots
½ medium red onion, cut into thin half-moons (about ½ cup)
1 small stalk celery, thinly sliced on a diagonal (about ¼ cup)
1 cucumber, unwaxed

- Place lettuce, carrot, onion, and celery in a serving bowl and toss to mix evenly. With a fork, make straight grooves down the skin of the cucumber, digging into skin only about ⅟₁₆ inch. Slice cucumber into thin rounds and mix in with other salad ingredients. Serve with Umeboshi-Sunflower Dressing (page 184).
- See also Hijiki Salad, page 173).

BEANS, BEAN PRODUCTS, AND SEA VEGETABLES

FRIED TEMPEH WITH GINGER

dark sesame oil
2 medium onions, cut into half-moons (about 2 cups)
1 pound tempeh, cut into 1 inch cubes
water
1 tablespoon juice from freshly grated ginger
tamari, to taste

• Heat a small amount of dark sesame oil in a skillet. Sauté onions for 2–3 minutes over fairly high flame, stirring constantly. Add tempeh and sauté for 1–2 minutes. Add enough water to half cover onions and tempeh; add ginger juice and cover skillet. Reduce flame to medium-low and cook for 25 minutes. Season with a small amount of tamari and simmer several minutes longer. Remove cover, turn flame up slightly, and cook until all water has evaporated. Mix onions and tempeh together and place in a serving bowl.

FRIED TOFU

1 pound fresh firm-style tofu
dark sesame oil
tamari, to taste
fresh parsley sprig, as garnish

• Slice tofu into pieces 3 inches long by 2 inches wide by ½ inch thick. Heat a small amount of dark sesame oil in a skillet. Set sliced tofu in skillet and pour 2–3 drops of tamari on top of each slice. Fry over medium-high flame for 2–3 minutes. Turn slices over and place 1–2 drops of tamari on top. Fry for 2–3 minutes. Turn over once more and fry for 1–2 minutes so that both sides are golden brown. Remove and arrange attractively on a platter. Garnish with a sprig of fresh parsley either in the center or off to one side of the platter.

BOILED TEMPEH AND SCALLIONS

1 pound tempeh
1 tablespoon finely chopped scallion roots (the white part
    and root hairs)
water
tamari, to taste
2 bunches scallions, sliced into 2-inch lengths (about 2 cups)

• Slice tempeh into pieces 2 inches long by 1 inch wide by ½ inch thick. Heat ¼ cup water in a skillet. Add scallion roots and water, and sauté over high flame for 2–3 minutes. Add tempeh and enough water to half cover tempeh. Bring to a boil. Cover, reduce flame to medium-low, and simmer for 25 minutes. Season with a little tamari, cover, and simmer for another 5 minutes or so. Add sliced scallions so that they sit on top of tempeh (do not mix). Cover and cook for 1–2 minutes, until scallions are tender and bright green. Remove cover, turn flame to high, and cook off any remaining liquid. Mix and place in a serving dish.

SCRAMBLED TOFU

dark sesame oil
1 cup diced onions
¼ cup sliced burdock, cut into matchsticks
1–2 medium carrots, cut into matchsticks (about ½ cup)
1 pound fresh tofu
tamari or sea salt, to taste
½ cup chopped parsley

• Heat a small amount of dark sesame oil in a skillet. Sauté onions over fairly high flame for 2–3 minutes. Layer burdock and carrots on top of onions. Crumble tofu on top. Cover, reduce flame to medium-low, and cook several minutes, until tofu is soft and fluffy and vegetables are tender. Season with a little tamari or sea salt and continue to cook, uncovered, until almost all liquid has evaporated. Mix in parsley and place in a serving bowl.

BROILED TOFU

1 pound fresh firm-style tofu
tamari, to taste

• Slice tofu into pieces 3 inches long by 2 inches wide by ½ inch thick. Place on a cookie sheet and put 2–3 drops of tamari on each slice. Place in the broiler and broil until golden brown. Turn slices over, put 1–2 drops of tamari on top, and place back in the broiler. Broil for 2–3 minutes, until tofu is golden brown and very soft. Remove and arrange attractively on a serving platter.

Adzuki Beans with Kombu and Squash

1 kombu strip, 6–8 inches long, soaked and cut into 1-inch squares
1 cup buttercup cubed squash *or* Hokkaido pumpkin, cut into
    2-inch chunks
1 cup adzuki beans, soaked 6–8 hours
water
sea salt, to taste

- Place kombu in a pot and set squash on top. Place adzuki beans on top of squash. Add just enough water to cover squash but not beans. Bring to a boil, cover, and reduce flame to medium-low. Simmer 1½–2 hours or until beans are fairly soft. Season with a little sea salt (¼ teaspoon per cup of beans at most). Simmer another half hour or until beans are very creamy and much of the remaining liquid is gone. Place in a serving bowl and serve.

Sea Vegetables

Hijiki Salad

water
2 cups soaked and sliced hijiki
several drops tamari
1 medium onion, cut into half-moons (about 1 cup)
½ cup carrots, cut into matchsticks (about ½ cup)
1–2 medium stalks celery, thinly sliced on a diagonal (about ½ cup)
¼ cup roasted sunflower seeds (page 191)

- Place about ½ inch of water in a saucepan and bring to a boil. Add hijiki and tamari. Cover saucepan, reduce flame to medium-low, and simmer for 15–20 minutes. Remove, drain, and place hijiki in a serving bowl.
- Place 1 inch of water in a pot and bring to a boil. Add onions and boil for 1 minute. Use a slotted spoon to remove onions, leaving the cooking water in the pot. Drain onions in a colander before placing in bowl with hijiki. Boil carrots in the same water for 1–2 minutes. Remove, drain, and place in bowl with hijiki and onions. Next boil celery in the same water for 1 minute. Remove, drain, and place in bowl with hijiki and vegetables. Mix thoroughly; add roasted sunflower seeds and mix again. Serve plain or with tofu or umeboshi dressing.

ARAME WITH CARROTS AND ONIONS

dark sesame oil
2 cups arame, washed and drained
1 medium onion, cut into half-moons (about 1 cup)
2–3 medium carrots, cut into matchsticks (about 1 cup)
water
tamari, to taste

- Heat a small amount of dark sesame oil in a skillet. Sauté arame for 2–3 minutes. Set onions and carrots on top of arame and add enough water to half cover arame. Add 3–4 drops of tamari, cover skillet, and reduce flame to medium-low. Simmer for about 25–30 minutes. Season with a little more tamari for a mild salt taste and continue cooking until all remaining liquid is gone. Place in a serving dish, and serve.

TOASTED NORI

1 sheet nori

- Turn flame to high. Hold nori sheet about 10 inches above flame with inside fold facing down (toward flame). Rotate nori sheet above flame until its color changes from black to bright green. Remove from flame.
- To make nori strips, cut toasted nori sheet crosswise. Cut each section crosswise again to create 4 large strips. Then, across the width of these large strips, cut thin strips about 2 inches long by ¼ inch wide.
- Serve toasted nori strips with grated daikon or mochi, or as a garnish for soups or noodles.

SOUPS

LENTIL SOUP

1 kombu strip, 6 inches long, soaked and cut into ½-inch squares
1 cup diced onions
1 cup diced celery
1 cup green lentils
5–6 cups water
sea salt
1 cup whole-wheat elbow noodles or shells
¼ cup chopped parsley, as garnish

- Place kombu, onions, celery, lentils, and water in a pot. Cover and bring to a boil. Reduce flame to medium-low and simmer for about 45 minutes. Season with a little sea salt, add the uncooked noodles, and simmer for several minutes more, uncovered, until noodles are tender. Place soup in individual serving bowls and garnish with a little chopped parsley.

CHICKPEA SOUP

1 cup chickpeas, soaked 6–8 hours
1 kombu strip, 6–8 inches long, soaked and cut into 1-inch squares
1 cup diced onions
5 cups water
sea salt, to taste
chopped scallions or parsley, as garnish

- Place chickpeas, kombu, and onions in a pressure cooker. Add water and place cover on pressure cooker. Turn flame to high and bring cooker up to pressure. Reduce flame to medium-low and cook for 1 hour.
- Remove cooker from flame and allow pressure to come down. Remove cover and season with a little sea salt for a mild taste. Simmer several minutes longer. Place soup in individual serving bowls and garnish with chopped scallions or parsley.

MISO SOUP

5 cups water
4–5 shiitake mushrooms, soaked, stems removed, and sliced
1 kombu strip, 6 inches long, soaked

4–5 teaspoons puréed barley (mugi) miso, or to taste

1 cup fresh snow peas, stems removed

- Place water, shiitake, and kombu in a pot and bring to a boil. Cover and reduce flame to medium-low. Simmer for about 10 minutes. Remove kombu, slice very thin, and place back in water. Reduce flame to very low, add puréed miso and snow peas, and simmer 2–3 minutes longer. Place soup in individual serving bowls, and serve.

FRENCH ONION SOUP

dark sesame oil

4–5 medium onions, thinly sliced on a diagonal (abour 4–5 cups)

4–5 shiitake mushrooms, soaked, stems removed, and sliced

5 cups water

tamari, to taste

2 slices whole-wheat sourdough bread, cut into 1-inch cubes,
   as garnish

¼ cup chopped scallions, chives, or parsley, as garnish

- Heat a small amount of dark sesame oil in a pot. Sauté onions for 3–4 minutes, until onions are translucent. Add sliced shittake mushrooms and sauté for another 1–2 minutes.
- Add water and bring to a boil. Cover pot and reduce flame to medium-low; simmer for 30 minutes or until onions are very soft. Season with a small amount of tamari for a mild-tasting soup.
- Heat 1 inch of sesame oil in a skillet. When oil is hot, add bread cubes and deep-fry until golden brown. Remove and drain on clean paper towels.
- Place soup in individual serving bowls and garnish each serving with sev-

eral deep-fried bread cubes and some chopped scallions, chives, or parsley. A few strips of toasted nori may be used in addition.

- Instead of bread cubes, you may use 1 inch squares of baked, toasted, or deep-fried mochi for garnish.

WATERCRESS SOUP

5 cups water

1 kombu strip, 4 inches long, soaked

4 shiitake mushrooms, soaked, stems removed, and sliced

½ cup tofu, sliced into ¼-inch cubes

4–5 teaspoons puréed barley (mugi) miso, or to taste

½ bunch of watercress

- Place water, kombu, and shiitake in a pot and bring to a boil. Cover and reduce flame to medium-low. Simmer for 10 minutes. Remove kombu and set aside for use in other dishes. Add tofu and miso, reduce flame to very low, and simmer for 2–3 minutes. Place 2–3 sprigs of watercress in each individual serving bowl and pour the hot soup over it. The heat from the soup will be enough to properly cook the watercress. Serve soup immediately after placing it in bowls.

PURÉED SQUASH SOUP

5–6 cups cubed buttercup squash *or* Hokkaido pumpkin

4–5 cups water

sea salt, to taste

¼ cup chopped scallions or parsley, as garnish

1 sheet nori, toasted and cut into thin strips (page 175), as garnish

- Place squash, water, and a small pinch of sea salt in a pot. Cover and bring to a boil. Reduce flame to medium-low and simmer for several minutes, until squash is very soft and tender. Place squash and cooking water in a hand food mill and purée to a smooth, creamy consistency. Return puréed squash to pot and bring back to a boil. Reduce flame to low, season with a little sea salt, and simmer for about 10 minutes. Place soup in individual serving bowls and garnish with chopped scallions or parsley and several strips of toasted nori.

Miso Soup with Wakame and Daikon

5 cups water
2 cups quartered and thinly sliced daikon, cut on a diagonal
3 shiitake mushrooms, soaked, stems removed, and sliced
¼ cup sliced wakame, washed and soaked
4–5 teaspoons puréed barley (mugi) miso, or to taste
¼ cup chopped scallions, as garnish

- Place water in a pot and bring to a boil. Add daikon and shiitake mushrooms. Reduce flame to medium-low, cover, and simmer for 3–5 minutes, until daikon is tender. Add wakame and simmer for 2–3 minutes longer. Reduce flame to very low, season with puréed miso for a mild taste, and simmer 2–3 minutes more. Place soup in individual serving bowls and garnish with chopped scallions.

SEITAN BARLEY SOUP

1 kombu strip, 4 inches long, soaked and cut into ½-inch squares

1 tablespoon finely chopped parsley stems or scallion roots (the white
    bottom part and root hairs)

¼ cup sliced shiitake or regular mushrooms

1 cup diced onions

¼ cup diced celery

½ cup diced carrots

¼ cup diced burdock

¼ cup barley, soaked 6–8 hours

1 cup cooked seitan, cut into 1-inch cubes (page 143)

5 cups water

tamari, to taste

¼ cup chopped parsley or scallions, as garnish

- Place kombu and parsley stems or scallion roots in a large pot. In order, layer shiitake, onions, celery, carrots, burdock, and barley on top. Place cooked seitan on top of barley. Add water and bring to a boil. Cover and reduce flame to medium-low. Simmer for about 1 hour, until barley is very soft. Season with a little tamari and continue to simmer over low flame until soup is very soft and creamy. Place soup in individual serving bowls and garnish with chopped parsley or scallions.

CLEAR BROTH

1 kombu strip, 4 inches long, soaked
5 cups water
1–2 medium stalks celery, thinly sliced on a diagonal (about ½ cup)
2 cups sliced Chinese cabbage, cut diagonally into 1-inch pieces
sea salt, to taste
chopped scallions, as garnish

- Place kombu and water in a pot and bring to a boil. Cover, reduce flame to medium-low, and simmer for about 10 minutes. Remove kombu and set aside for future use. Add celery and cook for 1 minute. Add Chinese cabbage and cook for 2 minutes. Season with a little sea salt and simmer 2 minutes more. Place broth in individual serving bowls and garnish with chopped scallions.

MISO-SQUASH SOUP

5 cups water
1 medium onion, cut into half-moons (about 1 cup)
2 cups cubed acorn squash, cut into 1-inch chunks
½ cup sliced wakame, washed and soaked
4–5 teaspoons puréed barley (mugi) miso, or to taste
¼ cup chopped scallions, as garnish

- Place water in a pot and bring to a boil. Add onions and squash. Cover pot and reduce flame to medium-low. Simmer for several minutes, until squash is tender. Add wakame and simmer for 2–3 minutes. Reduce flame to very low and add puréed miso for a mild taste. Place soup in individual serving bowls and garnish with chopped scallions.

SUPPLEMENTARY FOODS

Condiments

GOMASHIO

1⅓ tablespoons sea salt
1 cup black or tan sesame seeds

- Place sea salt in a stainless-steel skillet and roast over medium-low flame for several minutes, constantly stirring back and forth. Place sea salt in a suribachi and grind to a fine powder.
- Heat a dry stainless-steel skillet and place washed sesame seeds in it. Dry-roast seeds for several minutes, constantly stirring back and forth to roast evenly. When seeds give off a nutty fragrance and begin to pop, remove from flame and place in suribachi with ground sea salt. Grind in a slow circular motion until sesame seeds are about half crushed. Remove and allow to cool. When gomashio is cool, store in an airtight glass container. Sprinkle a small amount of this condiment on rice or other grain dishes.

NORI CONDIMENT

5 sheets nori
water to cover
tamari to cover

- Pull the nori apart into approximately 1-inch pieces and place in a saucepan. Pour a mixture of equal parts water and tamari over the nori to just cover it. Bring to a boil, reduce flame to low, cover, and simmer until most of the liquid is gone. Season with additional tamari to create a slightly salty taste. Serve each person 1–2 teaspoons of this condiment with rice or other grains.

Dressings, Butters, and Spreads

TOFU DRESSING

1 small onion, grated
¼ cup umeboshi vinegar *or* 4 umeboshi plums, pitted
1 pound fresh tofu, drained
1 tablespoon tamari
½ cup chopped scallions or chives
½ cup water

• Place onion and umeboshi vinegar or plums in a suribachi. (If you use plums, grind them to a smooth paste with the onion in a suribachi.) Purée tofu in a hand food mill. Place puréed tofu in suribachi and grind to a smooth consistency. Add tamari, scallions or chives, and water. Purée and place in an attractive serving dish. Place a tablespoon or so of dressing on top of Boiled Salad (page 166) or Hijiki Salad (page 173), or use as a spread on bread, crackers, or rice cakes.

Umeboshi-Sunflower Dressing

2 umeboshi plums, pitted
¼ cup chopped scallions or chives
½ cup water
¼ cup roasted sunflower seeds (page 191), chopped

- Place plums in a suribachi and grind to a smooth paste. Add scallions or chives and grind for 2 minutes. Add water and sunflower seeds. Mix and serve over your favorite salad.

Umeboshi-Scallion Dressing

3 umeboshi plums, pitted
4 tablespoons tahini
¼ cup chopped scallions
1¼ cups water

- Place umeboshi in a suribachi and grind to a smooth paste. Add tahini and grind again. Add scallions and water, mix to a smooth consistency, and serve over your favorite salad.

Umeboshi-Sesame Dressing

½ cup roasted sesame seeds (page 191)
¼ cup umeboshi vinegar
¾ cup water
¼ cup chopped scallions

- Place roasted sesame seeds in a suribachi and grind until half crushed. Add vinegar, water, and scallions. Grind for 1–2 minutes. Serve over your favorite salad.

Onion Butter

dark sesame oil
10 cups diced onions
pinch of sea salt
water

- Heat a small amount of dark sesame oil in a heavy pot. Sauté onions for several minutes over medium-low flame until they become translucent. Stir often to sauté onions evenly.
- Add a pinch of sea salt and just enough water to cover the top of the onions. Cover pot and bring water to a boil. Reduce flame to low and simmer for several hours so that the onions become dark brown and very sweet. There should not be any liquid left and the onions should be almost melted. If necessary, add very small amounts of water occasionally during the cooking process to keep onions from burning.

- When onion butter is ready, allow it to cool completely. Use immediately on bread or rice cakes, or place in a glass jar with a lid. Store either in the refrigerator or in a cool place.

Fish and Seafood

BAKED SOLE WITH RICE

dark sesame oil
1 cup diced onions
¼ cup diced celery
4 cups pressure-cooked or boiled brown rice
¼ cup chopped parsley
½ cup tamari
½ cup water
1 teaspoon freshly grated ginger
2–3 pounds fresh fillet of sole
chopped parsley, as garnish
several lemon wedges, as garnish

- Heat a small amount of dark sesame oil in a skillet. Sauté onions and celery for 2–3 minutes. Place sautéed vegetables in a bowl with rice and parsley, and mix well. Transfer mixture to a casserole dish.
- Mix tamari, water, and ginger together. Place sole in a shallow bowl or dish and pour tamari-water-ginger mixture over it. Let sole marinate for 30–45 minutes. Place marinated sole evenly on top of rice in casserole dish. Cover casserole and bake at 350°F for approximately 30 minutes or until fish becomes tender. Remove casserole cover and bake another 5 minutes. Sprinkle a little chopped parsley over fish and serve with several lemon wedges for garnish.

GINGER BROILED SCALLOPS

2 pounds fresh scallops
1 tablespoon freshly grated ginger
½ cup water
¼ cup tamari
⅛ cup sake (rice wine; optional)
2 fresh parsley sprigs, as garnish

• Clean scallops and place in a bowl. Mix ginger, water, tamari, and sake together and pour over scallops. Marinate for 15–20 minutes. Place marinated scallops on a baking sheet and broil for 5–10 minutes or until very tender. Do not broil too long, as they will become tough. Place broiled scallops in a serving dish and garnish with fresh parsley sprigs.

Desserts and Snacks

RAISIN-NUT COOKIES

3 cups rolled oats
¼ teaspoon sea salt
1½ cups whole-wheat pastry flour
1 cup raisins
½ cup chopped almonds
½ cup chopped walnuts
3 tablespoons corn oil
1 cup barley malt
1 cup water

- Mix rolled oats, sea salt, flour, raisins, and nuts together. Add oil and mix again. Add barley malt and mix thoroughly. Add water to make a thick batter. Place spoonfuls of batter about 1½ inches apart on oiled cookie sheets and press down to form cookies. If cookies are too thick, they will not cook thoroughly. Bake at 375°F for 25–30 minute, or until golden brown. This recipe will yield between 1 and 2 dozen cookies.

BLUEBERRY COUSCOUS CAKE

2½ cups apple juice or water
pinch of sea salt
½ cup raisins
2 cups couscous

TOPPING
1 cup water
¼ cup barley malt
pinch of sea salt
3 cups fresh blueberries
2–3 tablespoons kuzu, diluted in a few tablespoons of water

- Place apple juice or water in a pot. Add sea salt and raisins. Bring to a boil. Cover, reduce flame to medium-low, and simmer for about 10 minutes. Add couscous, cover, and simmer for 3–5 minutes. Turn off flame and let couscous sit, covered, for about 10 minutes. The heat in the pot will cook the couscous thoroughly. After 10 minutes or so, remove couscous and place it in a glass or ceramic cake pan.
- To make topping, place water, barley malt, sea salt, and blueberries in a saucepan and bring to a boil. Reduce flame to low and add diluted kuzu. Stir constantly to prevent lumping. Simmer for 2–3 minutes and remove from flame.

- Press couscous down firmly with a rice paddle before adding topping. Pour topping over cake, spreading blueberries evenly. Set aside and allow to cool before serving.

APPLESAUCE

2 cups water
8–10 apples, peeled and sliced
¼ cup barley malt (optional)
pinch of sea salt

- Place water, apples, barley malt (if desired) and sea salt in a pot and bring to a boil. Reduce flame to low and simmer until apples are soft. Purée apples and cooking water in a hand food mill. For sweeter applesauce, cook a little longer so that the sauce becomes thick. Applesauce cooked without barley malt makes a good breakfast dish.

STEWED PEARS

5–6 pears, sliced
pinch of sea salt
4 cups water
½ cup raisins
4–5 tablespoons kuzu, diluted in several tablespoons of water

- Place pears, salt, water, and raisins in a pot and bring to a boil. Reduce flame to low and cover pot. Simmer for several minutes, until pears are soft. Add diluted kuzu, stirring to prevent lumping. Simmer 2–3 minutes and serve.

Apple-Raisin Kanten

4 apples, sliced
1 quart apple juice
pinch of sea salt
½ cup raisins
5–6 tablespoons agar-agar flakes

- Place apples, apple juice, salt, and raisins in a pot. Stir in agar-agar flakes and bring to a boil. Reduce flame to low and simmer for several minutes, until apples are soft. Pour liquid and apples into a dish or mold. Refrigerate or keep in a cool place until jelled. This will take about an hour or so. If the kanten is hard, slice into squares and serve. If it has a softer consistency, spoon into individual dessert bowls.

Couscous Cake with Pear Sauce

2½ cups apple juice
pinch of sea salt
2 cups couscous

TOPPING
5–6 pears, peeled and sliced
pinch of sea salt
1 cup water

- Place apple juice and a pinch of sea salt in a pot and bring to a boil. Reduce flame to low and add couscous. Cover and simmer for 2–3 minutes. Turn off flame and let couscous sit, covered, for several minutes.

- Place couscous in a glass or ceramic cake pan and press down firmly and evenly.
- To make pear sauce for topping, place pears, salt, and water in a pot and bring to a boil. Reduce flame, cover, and simmer for 4–5 minutes, until pears are soft. Purée in a hand food mill. Slice cake and spoon pear sauce over it while serving.

ROASTED NUTS AND TAMARI-ROASTED NUTS

- Raw almonds, walnuts, peanuts, and chestnuts are especially good roasted in the shell. Place whole nuts on a cookie sheet and roast in a 350°F oven for 10–12 minutes. If you use shelled nuts, they will cook faster.
- To make tamari-roasted nuts, simply sprinkle a mixture of equal parts tamari and water over shelled nuts toward the end of cooking.

ROASTED SEEDS

- Wash tan or black sesame seeds, hulled sunflower seeds, squash seeds, or green pumpkin seeds. Heat a skillet and dry-roast each variety separately over medium-low flame. Stir constantly to prevent burning and to roast seeds evenly.
- Tan sesame seeds and sunflower seeds will turn golden brown and begin to pop after 5 minutes or so; pumpkin seeds are ready when they turn golden brown. Season seeds with a small amount of tamari, if desired.
- Fresh acorn squash seeds can be roasted in the oven like nuts. They will turn golden brown.

ROASTED GRAINS AND BEANS

- Brown rice, sweet brown rice, barley, and rye can be dry-roasted for use as a snack. Soak grains for 24 hours prior to roasting. Heat a dry skillet and separately roast each type of grain until it turns golden brown and releases a nutty fragrance. Stir constantly to keep grain from burning. Wheatberries may be roasted the same way for use in recipes such as Pressure-Cooked Brown Rice and Wheatberries (page 133), but they are not generally recommended as a snack food.
- Dry-roasted black soybeans make a particularly good snack. Soak soybeans for 4–6 hours and dry-roast as described above. They are ready when the skins start to split and the beans are brown inside. While the beans are very hot, stir in a few drops of tamari, if desired, and continue cooking until the moisture steams off. Dried green peas may be dry-roasted the same way; they are ready when the skin begins to split and the peas are thoroughly heated.
- Roasted chickpeas, adzuki beans, and other beans are not generally recommended as a snack, as they can be difficult to digest, but they can be ground for use in homemade grain coffee.

Beverages

BANCHA TEA

1 quart water
1–2 tablespoons bancha twigs

- Place water and twigs in a teapot and bring to a boil. Reduce flame to low and simmer for 5–10 minutes. For milder-tasting tea, simmer for 3–4 minutes. Children may enjoy tea brewed to this strength. For stronger tea, simmer for 10–15 minutes. Bancha tea is good any time of day, but especially after meals.

GRAIN COFFEE

1 teaspoon prepared grain coffee
1 cup boiling water

- Prepared grain coffee is available at most natural foods stores. Place 1 teaspoon in a cup and pour hot water over it. Stir and drink. If you use homemade grain coffee, adjust the amounts to taste.

Amasake Drink

Amasake
4 cups sweet brown rice
8 cups water
½ cup koji
⅛ teaspoon sea salt

- Wash sweet rice and soak overnight in 8 cups of water. Place rice and water in a pressure cooker. Place cover on pressure cooker, turn flame to high, and bring the cooker up to pressure. Reduce the flame to medium-low, place a flame deflector under the cooker, and pressure-cook for 30 minutes. Remove cooker from flame and allow pressure to come down. Let rice cool for 45 minutes.
- Place rice in a glass bowl and mix in koji. Cover with a clean towel and set aside to ferment for 6–8 hours. Stir several times during the fermentation process to make sure the koji dissolves.
- Place fermented rice in a pot. Add sea salt and bring to a boil (boiling stops the fermentation process). As soon as mixture starts to bubble, remove from flame and allow to cool.
- Store amasake in a covered glass jar in the refrigerator. Use as a sweetener or in making Amasake Drink. For variety, you may use brown rice, millet, or barley in this recipe.

Amasake Drink
½ cup amasake
½ cup water

- Place amasake and water in a blender and blend to a creamy consistency. Amasake drink may be served hot with ginger, or with a teaspoon of grain coffee stirred in. It can also be enjoyed cool.

THIRTEEN

At Home
and on the Road

Eating at restaurants, entertaining, and traveling can be a healthful and enjoyable part of the macrobiotic lifestyle. This chapter offers a number of practical ideas that will help you in following the macrobiotic diet wherever you may be.

Chances are that there is a meal for you in the kitchen of any restaurant if you know how to ask for it. "Without cheese," "no dressing," "meatless," "no sauce," and "broiled or steamed instead of fried" are all increasingly common requests these days. You can ask your waiter or waitress to tell you about ingredients, additives, and the way the food is cooked before you place your order. After all, you are paying for your meal, and restaurateurs want their customers to be happy. Be creative and bold enough to ask for what you want, and your meal will probably exceed your expectations.

Unfortunately, most restaurants use sugar, common salt, black pepper, eggs, cheese, milk, and a number of chemical additives in their dishes. Certainly many cafeterias, fast-food establishments, "family" restaurants, and even some so-called health-food eateries are not the best choices. A local ethnic restaurant where some vegetarian foods are served is probably your best bet—unless, of course, there is a macrobiotic restaurant in your area, or a natural foods restaurant that serves macrobiotic dishes.

At Italian restaurants, soup, vegetables, pasta, salad, and baked or broiled fish are usually available without meat or tomato sauce. Most Chinese and Japanese restaurants serve steamed fish, vegetables, and rice. Requests for brown rice and "no MSG" can usually be accommodated.

Seafood restaurants are good too, especially if they serve freshly caught fish and cook it without too many trimmings. Fried fish, along with other fried foods, are best avoided, because restaurants generally use lard (animal fat) for frying. With dinner in a seafood restaurant, you can usually get rice or salad and cooked vegetables.

Greek, Middle Eastern, Indian, and Mexican restaurants usually serve one or more vegetarian grain and bean dishes. But in the case of the latter two, make sure you ask them to forgo use of chili or curry, if possible. In any restaurant, it is best to make sure that vegetable oils, not lard, are used in cooking.

ENTERTAINING

When you prepare a full-course macrobiotic meal for friends, it will most certainly be tasty and healthful. Start with an appetizer, and follow with soup or salad. Serve fish with whole grains and vegetables for an entrée. Dessert can be a piece of Couscous Cake with Pear Sauce. Bancha tea or grain coffee will complete the meal.

If you plan to dine with friends, you may want to tell them you don't eat meat, and perhaps offer to bring some home-cooked food for them to enjoy.

BRINGING LUNCH TO WORK

People who work outside the home frequently eat lunch out on weekdays. If you can find a restaurant where you can go for an occasional macrobiotic or natural-foods lunch, you are fortunate. Nevertheless, on a day-to-day-basis, it is best to bring lunch to work with you.

Macrobiotic meals are quite portable. If you buy a one- or two-cup size wide-mouth insulated container such as a thermos, you can transport whole grains, soups, stews, and beans. If these are warmed before you leave for work, the container will keep them warm. You may also choose to bring rice balls, cooked vegetables, salad, pickles, and a dessert such as granola or couscous cake. In addition, you may wish to bring in a snack such as rice cakes, raisins, dried apples, or roasted nuts or seeds, along with an insulated container of bancha tea.

Tasty and convenient sandwiches may be made with seitan, tempeh, or tofu and sliced cooked vegetables on sourdough or pita bread, with lettuce and pickles. The idea is to include some kind of whole grain, as well as something raw or pickled to lighten the meal. Leftovers from dinner the night before make especially good lunch meals. You may also want to get a teapot to brew fresh bancha tea at the office.

IN THE AIR

Many airlines have been scaling back their food offerings. However, if you will be on a longer flight with meal service, you can usually order the type of food you want on board by calling at least a day in advance of your flight. You may be able to order brown rice, miso soup, a bean dish, oatmeal, wild rice, or steamed vegetables. Beware of the "standard" vegetarian meal, as it usually comes filled with eggs, salt, and sugar, all floating in butter and topped with cheese. Your best bet is to call ahead to find out exactly what's available.

Just in case of a mishap, you can bring along a travel bag with an assortment of homemade sushi, rice balls, steamed and pickled vegetables, sourdough bread, powdered miso soup (available packaged—just pour the contents into a cup of hot water), and maybe a few homemade cookies and some bancha teabags.

It is a good idea to eat less than usual during travel. You will have more energy when you arrive at your destination and you will feel better, too.

ON THE ROAD

When you travel by car, you have more control over your food. If you bring a small cutting board, a sharp knife, several bowls, utensils, a small gas cooker (the type designed for camping, with two burners), two or three pots, a couple of wooden spoons, and a cooler chest with refreezable ice cubes (these can be placed in a motel ice chest if you stop overnight), you won't have to dine out at all. For food, you will need some quick-cooking grains such as roasted rice or barley, rice cream couscous, cornmeal, bulghur, and oatmeal; lentils, adzuki, split peas, and other quick-cooking beans; and sea vegetables, miso, tamari soy sauce, noodles, bancha tea, snacks, sourdough bread, and tortillas. You can store fresh vegetables and fruits, fish, amasake, tofu, tempeh, and other staples in a cooler and replenish supplies along the way. If you're planning to stop at motels, try to get a unit with a kitchen so that you can thoroughly clean all of your equipment, make some rice balls, bake some bread, and prepare a meal or two.

If you plan to be on the road for an extended journey, prepare ahead of time by doing some research into natural-foods stores and restaurants along your route. If you are in a city or town, you can always look in the Yellow Pages under "health" to find suppliers of natural and macrobiotic foods. In many cases, local restaurants will also be listed. If not, call one of the health-food stores in the area and ask if they can recommend a local restaurant.

Spending a little extra time in preparation will make the trip smoother, keep you healthier, and save you money. Of course, you may have to go out of your way a bit to find alternatives, but as so many people have discovered, you will probably meet others with common interests, sample some tasty vegetarian meals, and stock up on supplies. When you return home, you will know that it was worth it.

FOURTEEN

The Joy of Exercise

Walking, our natural means of transport, is an excellent form of exercise. Other exercises are used to produce specific results, as every individual has specific exercise needs. The exercise program we suggest, combined with the macrobiotic diet and a busy and active life, will improve cardiovascular health and normalize the flow of energy in the body.

The routine offers the same positive results as many common exercise programs such as calisthenics, weight training, and aerobics. The benefits are increased flexibility, endurance, and muscle tone; healthier blood; and weight loss. But the exercises presented here are superior because they work on all the major body systems rather than on a select few. Actually, the real focus of these exercises is on the internal workings of the body—the glands, organs, and overall metabolism. They are adapted from the centuries-old practice of *do-in*, a form of exercise and self-massage that promotes rejuvenation and longevity.

Many exercise programs concentrate on the external muscles while any internal benefits are secondary. You will certainly shape up performing the exercises that follow, but more important, you will be balancing and normalizing the flow of energy inside your body. In addition, you will be recharging your nervous system and your body's energy focal point located just below the navel. As this center of energy becomes charged, your level of physical and mental energy will surge.

After just a few weeks of daily exercise, your breathing will be freer, your muscles will be more toned, you will have more energy, and your appetite for more wholesome foods will increase.

The stretching movements will add flexibility and strength; at the same time, they will help you to develop the capacity for deep muscle relaxation. In time, your posture will also improve, your need for sleep will decrease, and your physical endurance and powers of concentration will increase. In other words, you will begin to experience what health really is—the joy of being alive and well.

By improving breathing capacity and circulation, exercise helps cleanse the blood. The added oxygen in the blood oxidizes (burns) impurities, and the lymphatic system, which carries wastes from the cells, also cleanses itself.

The added oxygen intake from exercise stimulates an increase in the basal metabolic rate, the rate at which the body uses energy when at rest. An increase in basal metabolic rate, along with increased activity, is an important factor in controlling weight, as it means that the body is burning food energy (calories) more rapidly.

Whether you begin the exercises when you are healthy or unwell, you will probably start to notice improvements after the first few sessions. *It is important, however, not to overdo it in the beginning, especially if you haven't exercised in some time.* To minimize the risk of your overdoing the exercises presented here, we suggest a one-minute rest period between the exercises. If you are not sure how much exercise is too much, try shortened movements and lengthened rest pauses between exercises. Don't extend your body beyond its present limits by holding on to your legs or feet if this causes pain. The movements aren't a test of flexibility, but rather a way to gradually improve it.

Check with your physician before beginning any exercise program if you have a history of heart problems or other physical restrictions. If you experience any sudden pains, cramps, or aches, slow down or stop exercising until they go away.

If you use a wheelchair or are confined to bed, even gentle or subtle movements may aid your body's healing efforts.

MERIDIAN STRETCHES

The following exercise routine will take between twenty and forty minutes to perform depending upon your energy level and desire. Its primary emphasis is upon the system of meridians described by modern acupuncture theory. There are fourteen meridians (lines of energy flow) that run up and down the body, extending to both internal organs and external body parts, including the toes, hands, face, and scalp. According to Oriental medicine, if the electromagnetic energy flow through the meridians is harmonious and free, the person is healthy. The meridian stretches help to reestablish and maintain a balanced energy flow. While performing the routine, imagine clear and unblocked energy flowing through each meridian as described in the captions beneath Figures 14.1 through 14.7. Such a positive mental focus will enhance the effectiveness of the stretches.

Use the routine once a day, in the morning or evening, or whenever you can find the time. Keep in mind that it is better to do the exercises at least every other day than it is to miss several days in a row.

When exercising, hold each of the positions at their point of extension for one full breath, then revert to the original position, and rest for about thirty seconds before moving on to the next stretching movement. Also, in all of the movements, bend from the waist rather than from your upper back. The point of extension will be different for each person; the distance you can stretch is not nearly so important as performing the exercise with correct form.

When you complete an exercise, *be sure to pause for a full minute before moving on to the next exercise.* In a twenty-minute routine, this will cut the actual exercise time to about fifteen minutes—with five minutes of rest to allow your body to prepare for the next exercise.

Trunk Bend

Standing with your feet shoulders' width apart, clasp your hands behind your back. Slowly bend forward, raising your arms behind you and keeping the hands clasped. Bend from the waist as far forward and as far down as possible, extending the hands beyond the line of the head, as shown in Figure 14.1. Take a full breath and slowly return to the original standing position. Pause briefly and repeat the movement, a dozen times in all. Rest for a minute and move to the next exercise.

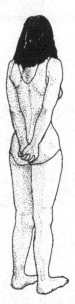

(a) Starting position

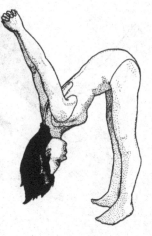

(b) Extension

Figure 14.1   Trunk Bend
This exercise stimulates the lung and large intestine meridians, which run along the outside of the arm and hand.

Alternate Leg Stretch

Sit with both legs extended in front of you, opened as widely as possible. Reach forward with both arms extended toward your right foot, making sure the knees are locked with the backs of the legs close to or touching the floor. As shown in Figure 14.2, bend the entire trunk of your body from the waist, letting your head drop as you stretch. When you reach the point of extension, take a full breath. Slowly return to the original sitting position. Turn and repeat the same movement toward the opposite leg. Pause for a breath before repeating. Keep alternating until you have stretched in each direction six times. Stand and rest for a minute, then move on to the next exercise.

Front Body Stretch

Sit on the floor with your legs folded to the sides as shown in Figure 14.3, and place a pillow or two behind your buttocks. Slowly and carefully bend back-

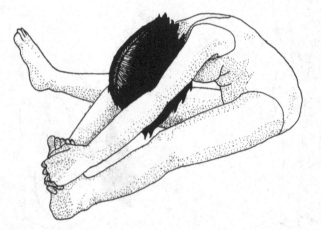

Figure 14.2   Alternate Leg Stretch
This exercise stimulates the liver and gallbladder meridians. The liver meridian runs along the inside of the leg to the torso. The gallbladder meridian passes along the leg, over the torso, under the arm from front to back, and over the shoulder, extending up to the temple.

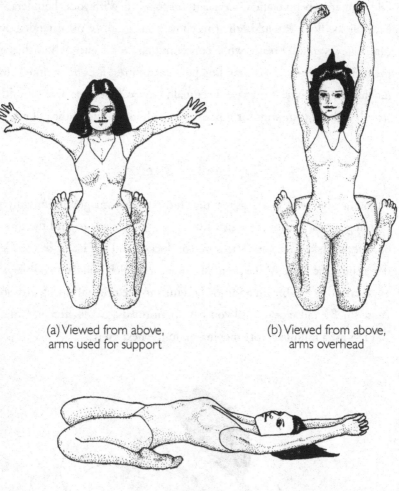

(a) Viewed from above, arms used for support

(b) Viewed from above, arms overhead

(c) Side view

Figure 14.3   Front Body Stretch
This exercise stimulates the stomach meridian and the spleen-pancreas meridian.
The stomach meridian runs up the front leg, across the torso, ending on the face.
The spleen-pancreas meridian runs up the inside of the leg and over the chest,
ending under the arm.

ward, lowering your shoulders and back to the floor. If this is too difficult, fold your arms behind and underneath for support. With your shoulders and back on the floor, extend both arms above your head. In the extended posture, take seven full breaths while concentrating on the energy flow through the meridians. Return to a standing position and rest for one minute before moving on to the next exercise. Eventually, you will become able to do this stretch without your arms for support and without the aid of the pillows.

Double Leg Stretch

Sit on the floor with your legs together and extended straight in front of you. Bending forward from the waist, reach with your hands toward the toes of both feet. Make sure your knees remain locked and the backs of your legs rest against the floor. At the point of extension, which is illustrated in Figure 14.4, take one full breath and slowly return to the original sitting position. Pause briefly and repeat until you have performed a dozen stretches. Stand and rest for a minute before moving on to the next exercise.

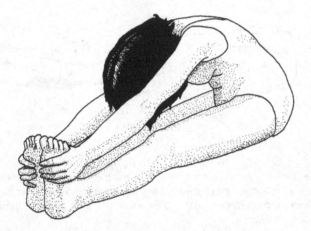

Figure 14.4   Double Leg Stretch
This exercise stimulates the kidney and bladder meridians. The kidney meridian runs
up the back of the leg and around the body, ending on the chest. The bladder
meridian runs down the back of the torso and leg.

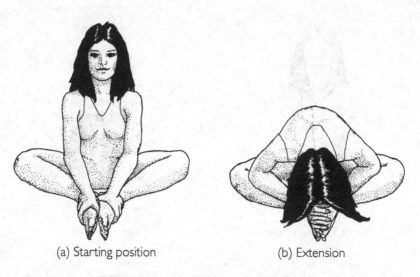

(a) Starting position   (b) Extension

Figure 14.5   Open Leg Bend
This exercise stimulates the heart and small intestine meridians. The heart meridian
runs up the arm, ending under the armpit, and the small intestine meridian runs
up the back of the arm, ending on the face.

Open Leg Bend

Sit on the floor with your legs open in front of you, soles of the feet together, and knees wide apart. Holding your toes with both hands, slowly bend forward from the waist, bringing your nose toward the arches of the feet (see Figure 14.5). At the point of extension, take a full breath and return to the original sitting position. Pause briefly and repeat until you have performed a dozen bends. Stand and rest for a minute before moving on to the next exercise.

Crossover Bend

Sit on the floor with your ankles crossed close to the body and knees wide apart. Also cross your arms in front so that the right hand grasps the left knee, and the left hand the right knee. Now bend forward from the waist as far as you can, trying to touch your forehead to the floor in front of you. At the point of extension, which is illustrated in Figure 14.6, take a full breath

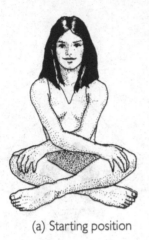

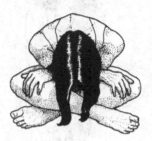

(a) Starting position   (b) Extension

Figure 14.6   Crossover Bend
This exercise stimulates the two comprehensive circulatory meridians, which are
known as the triple heater (TH) and the governing vessel (GV). The TH runs
along the middle of the inside and outside of the arm; the GV passes up and
down the front and back of the torso from the groin to the buttocks.

and return to the original cross-legged sitting position. Pause briefly and repeat until you have performed twelve stretches. Stand and rest for a minute
before moving on to the side stretch.

Side Stretch

Stand with your feet at the width of one and a half shoulders apart, hands
extended straight above your head, and thumbs (but not hands) clasped together. Bend from the waist to the left side until your trunk and arms are at
a ninety-degree angle to the floor, as shown in Figure 14.7. At the point of
extension, twist your trunk so that you are now looking toward the ground,
keeping thumbs clasped and arms extended outward as far as possible. Hold
the position for a full breath. Rotate the trunk again, slowly returning to the
original position. Pause and repeat the exercise to the left side, and then alternate right and left sides until you have performed the movement six times
on each side.

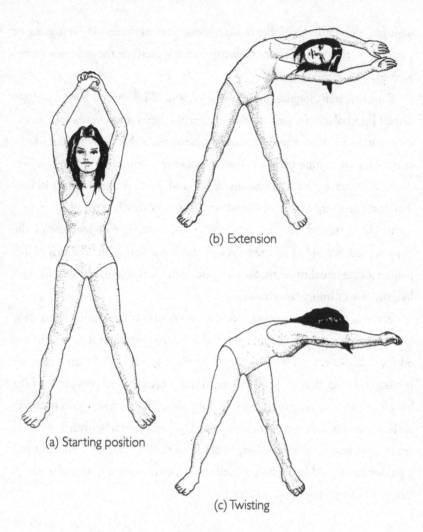

(a) Starting position

(b) Extension

(c) Twisting

Figure 14.7   Side Stretch
This exercise stimulates many of the meridians simultaneously.

WALKING

Many people take up running or jogging for exercise. Perhaps one reason that jogging has become so popular is that it balances a high-fat diet. It helps to develop extra routes of circulation for blood to flow through, while a high-fat, high-cholesterol diet tends to close normal routes off. So jogging or running increases circulatory capacity and may reduce the risks associated with eating the modern diet.

Unfortunately, jogging has drawbacks, too. While over a period of time it may be a balancing form of exercise for the heart and circulation, in the short run, it tends to unevenly stress the heart and other body parts and systems. Although some people can enjoy jogging or running, joggers are frequently halted by back problems, bone and joint disorders, and kidney damage, due to the shock of pounding up and down while running.

In the words of Thomas Jefferson, "The sovereign invigorator of the body is exercise, and of all the exercises walking is best." The rewards of just plain walking equal those that can be obtained from any other exercise, with half the risk of injury or exhaustion.

If you are like many people today, however, you can probably think of at least five reasons why you couldn't put this book down right this minute and take a walk—it's too dark out, there's no place to walk, there isn't time, it's raining, it's cold, and so on. It is easy to make excuses, but you can't get the benefits of an exercise program by reading about it. You have to do it. Safety is always a consideration, but during the day, parks and schoolyards are generally good places for a refreshing walk. If it's raining, put on a raincoat and a pair of boots and bring an umbrella. If it's cold, wear a coat and a hat. A half hour of walking per day helps to:

- Control your weight by increasing your basal metabolic rate;
- Improve blood circulation and quality, warming the hands and feet;
- Prevent heart problems and other illnesses;
- Aid digestion and elimination;
- Act as a mild appetite suppressant;
- Keep bones healthy and strong;
- Relieve tension and worry;
- Prevent respiratory disorders;
- Burn off fat;

- Tone muscles, especially thighs, calves, and hips; and
- Improve appearance.

Some exercise physiologists consider walking to be a "second heart" because during walking the muscles of the feet, calves, thighs, buttocks, and abdomen rhythmically contract and release. So does the diaphragm, the powerful muscle that is part of our breathing apparatus. As the muscles contract and release, they squeeze the veins, pressing the blood upward toward the heart.

If you do not walk, your blood tends to pool in the belly, hips, thighs, and feet. Circulation slows, and the heart must work harder to make sure that enough oxygen reaches the cells and that wastes are removed. When you stand still or sit for long periods of time, your brain also suffers from a lack of oxygen.

To begin a walking program, all you need is a comfortable pair of shoes. Running shoes are especially good. For maximum benefit, your stride should be brisk. Let your arms swing freely at your sides and keep your head up. Rhythm is the key.

Try to find a place to walk where you can establish a steady pace without a lot of starts and stops. If possible, avoid crowded sidewalks and noisy or heavily trafficked avenues, and find a park, a trail in the woods, or a beach. Walking barefoot on the grass or on a beach is the most invigorating of all.

SOME ADDITIONAL TIPS

Make it a priority to walk every day, for it is important to make time to do the things that will benefit your health.

The morning is the best time to walk. Many of the most confident, relaxed, and content people have learned to begin their day with light exercise and a walk. The air seems fresher and the activity seems to awaken and stimulate physical and mental processes that otherwise remain half asleep. Scientists explain this phenomenon by pointing to endorphins, brain chemicals that are released by physical activities such as a good walk. If scientists have discovered anything that could be called "happy" chemicals, they would be the endorphins. A brisk morning walk is much better than a cup of coffee for "starting your engine."

It will benefit your health and the environment if you start your *own* engine instead of driving your car for every little errand. When you must drive, park in the space farthest from the store rather than the closest. Walk to work. Get a dog and let him walk you if you won't take yourself out. As long as you stay warm and dry, a walk in rain or snow will leave you feeling vitalized.

A half hour each day is a good amount of time to spend walking. A full hour every other day is also fine. Whatever you do, don't overdo it. Especially if you are ill, convalescent, or out of shape, start out slowly, walking no more than is comfortable. Every few days increase the distance by 10 to 20 percent.

Ideally, before you head out to walk, perform either the stretches presented in this chapter or other light stretching exercises. If you feel too stiff and a little sleepy in the morning, get out and walk first and do the stretches when you return. Follow your morning exercise session with one of the macrobiotic breakfast dishes in the recipe section.

Walking and stretching, together with a wholesome diet, are important aspects of the macrobiotic way. Many people have found health and happiness in these simple principles.

FIFTEEN

Improving Your Overall Quality of Life

B y becoming more aware of the factors that affect the quality of life, we can improve it. So far we have discussed the roles of diet and exercise in improving physical health. In this chapter, we will discuss the effects of diet, attitude, and environment on the quality of life.

The macrobiotic philosophical, social, and biological views have direct practical application. The following suggestions for reducing the day-to-day stresses we all encounter are called *general lifestyle suggestions* and *daily reflections*. The first group has to do with our habits in eating, personal hygiene, and living; the second, with our thoughts and attitudes about life.

GENERAL LIFESTYLE SUGGESTIONS

The suggestions that follow aren't hard and fast rules, but neither are they intended to be taken lightly. For as scientists learn more about many of our modern inventions and conveniences, such as microwave ovens, television, and chemical-laden "body-care" products, more warnings are being placed on more packages, and it is up to the educated and aware consumer to avoid the dangers. Beginning with eating patterns, I will offer some alternatives to several questionable and quite possibly detrimental habits that many of us have fallen into.

Do you drink only when you're thirsty and eat only when hungry? Probably not. Most of us eat and drink too often and too much. The result is fatigue and a widespread problem of obesity. How do you know when you're hungry? It is basically a question of sensitivity. By eating macrobiotically, you'll find that two to three well-balanced meals, including soup, and two or three cups of tea daily satisfy hunger and thirst. Of course your needs will depend on your level of activity and the other factors mentioned in Chapter 1. As long as the meals are properly balanced, you may eat as much as you want (short of stuffing yourself full at each meal). If several hours elapse between meals, you may want to have a snack as well.

Regardless of how much you eat, make sure to chew each bite of food thoroughly. By chewing each bite of food until liquefied, you mix it with digestive enzymes, which are especially important for the proper digestion of complex carbohydrates—the major nutrients in the macrobiotic diet.

Another general suggestion on the matter of eating is to stop late-night snacking. Eating less than an hour or so before bed is unhealthful for two reasons: First, you can't sleep soundly while your belly is full of food; and second, you can't digest food properly while your body is half asleep. The result is stagnation in the intestines and a less than adequate night's rest.

In addition to changing eating habits, there are other ways to reduce day-to-day stress.

One of these ways is to sleep soundly and peacefully. To achieve this, I recommend that you retire before midnight as often as possible and wake up around sunrise. Sleep researchers have determined that we get our most regenerating rest between 9:00 P.M. and 1:00 A.M.

For personal hygiene, it is preferable to wash your skin with pure soap and to minimize the use of chemically produced body-care products. Most commercial cosmetics and detergent or deodorant soaps are damaging to the healthy bacteria on the skin. After lathering up with soap, it takes one to four hours and plenty of vitamin C to replace the so-called "acid mantle" that protects the skin. It is best to use small quantities of pure soap under the arms, around the genitals, and on the face, hands, and feet—and as shampoo. On the rest of the body, use a hot, damp washcloth or loofah sponge and rub vigorously instead. This will stimulate healthy blood circulation to the skin and better elimination through the pores. Avoid taking lengthy hot baths or showers.

In addition, try replacing commercial cosmetics with the natural products available in natural foods stores. For example, you may want to use sesame or peanut oil as a moisturizer, oatmeal or clay as a facial pack, herbal teas for a facial steam, and lemon juice or cider vinegar diluted with water as an astringent.

All fabrics used close to the skin ought to be as natural as possible. Try to gradually shift from nonabsorbent synthetic-fiber clothes to more comfortable and absorbent cotton, linen, silk, or wool clothing.

Around your home, try to replace synthetic towels, sheets, blankets, and carpets with natural-fiber ones. Incandescent full-spectrum lighting is better than fluorescent lights, and wooden furniture also contributes to a more healthful atmosphere. House plants freshen and oxygenate the air inside your home, contributing to a cheerful, relaxed environment.

Even in the winter, it is a good idea, occasionally, to open windows to permit fresh air to circulate. During colder weather, try not to keep your home overly warm. A slightly cool indoor temperature will help your body adapt better to the cold outdoors. In summer, try using a fan rather than air conditioning. Let your internal bodily thermostat take over from the one on the wall.

Planting a vegetable garden in the springtime is a wonderful thing. Learning to grow and harvest your own food is a rewarding experience. The soil is life itself, and spending time building it and nurturing plants as they grow can transfer that life to your body. If you don't have space to grow vegetables, try flowers.

A number of the modern convenience items many of us take for granted, such as hair dryers, electric toothbrushes, and microwave ovens, may not be good for our health. Modern testing instruments and biofeedback have shown that virtually all electrical appliances sap human energy when they are operated close to the body for extended periods of time. Appliances produce positive ions, which carry an electrical charge opposite to the ions created by growing plants, a waterfall, or rain. Negative ions are known to have a calming effect. Exposure to positive ions from fluorescent lighting, or from sitting in front of electric and electronic machines all day long, may be harmful. If your work demands that you expose yourself to positive ionization, that is all the more reason to avoid it at home.

Another item almost everyone takes for granted is the television set. Color sets especially have been known to emit low-level radiation. The best way to protect yourself from potential harm is, of course, by avoiding television. The next best thing is to watch it at a distance of about fifteen feet.

Macrobiotics doesn't favor a return to some past way of life. It appreciates, values, and continues to use some of the technological advances of modern society. However, many home appliances and cooking devices are unnecessary, and artificially and synthetically produced goods may contribute to the development of illness.

DAILY REFLECTIONS

These daily reflections are suggestions for ways of thinking in tune with nature and with good health. At first it will be helpful to set aside a few minutes each day to ponder the ideas. In time, you will find yourself being reminded of these calming thoughts no matter where you are or what you are doing.

The first idea is simply to appreciate nature. The way you do this is up to you. You may take a walk in the woods, paint a picture of a tree, write a poem, or sit outside on the porch. Whatever you do, try to leave the cares of your day behind. There will be plenty of time to work them out later. Let this brief period be only for you and thoughts of nature.

Changing the way you eat, dress, and live tends to keep you focused for a time on the reasons why you are making these changes. While it is important to be focused on your new directions, try to avoid being preoccupied with the state of your health. Keep active physically and mentally.

Try to encourage family members, especially your spouse, to make positive living changes with you. Unfortunately, not everyone receives the support of a spouse, family, or friends in their wish to eat macrobiotically. Understand that those close to you want the best for you, regardless of how it seems. The best way to gain the support of others is to give them yours. Show them that you care about them and they will do the same for you.

Be grateful for all you have, for your grandparents and their parents who made it possible for you and your parents to be here. If you have the inclination, reconstruct your family tree. Find out how far back you can trace your roots. Most libraries have books that can help you do this.

At mealtimes, be thankful for your food and the company you have to share it with. Let the thanks come from a place deep inside you. A moment of silence or a short prayer before meals gives you an opportunity to slow down, while your body prepares itself for the food. It is the best time to let go of all the worries and responsibilities that can interrupt smooth digestion.

Finally, the expression "one grain, ten thousand grains" relates a great truth of nature. For every seed of wheat given to the earth at planting time, the earth eventually returns ten thousand, even ten million, at the harvest. In the same way, share the love and energy you receive to help others achieve better health and happiness. Teaching others is the best way to learn something for yourself. By teaching them about macrobiotics, you will fortify it in yourself.

The lifestyle suggestions and daily reflections can help you along the road to self-discovery, self-knowledge, and better health, improving not only the quality of your own life, but increasing the happiness and joy of those around you.

Beating Diabetes: Larry Bogoslaw's Story

I had always liked sweets, and I had a problem with bedwetting since I was four, but I never had any real problems with my health until one October, when I was eight years old. I remember the night of my cousin's bar mitzvah: I hadn't eaten all day, and I was so hungry by the end of the evening that I binged on as much cake as I could eat. The next morning I threw up and began to feel really fatigued. My mother took me to a pediatrician, and the diagnosis was type 1 diabetes; I was put on one shot of insulin per day.

I lacked the willpower to stay on the structured diet plan I was given. By the time I was eleven, another doctor put me on two shots of insulin a day in an effort to better control my blood sugar, since I wasn't eating as carefully as I was supposed to. From the start, I was always a very undisciplined eater and drinker, and very poor at following any doctor's instructions; in fact, developing the ability to be orderly and disciplined in my approach to taking care of myself has been one of the biggest changes I have experienced now in my year of practicing macrobiotics. I recall always being angry in the first few years. I had cut sugar out of my diet, but I was still eating plenty of meat.

When I was sixteen, my father discovered macrobiotics in Philadelphia through the East West Foundation. Although my father began eating macrobiotically, I didn't begin until I went to Boston in June three years later, where I had my first macrobiotic consultation and was given a completely different way to eat right away. At this time I was taking 65 units of insulin a day. Marc Van Cauwenberghe, the consultant I saw, told me I could possibly be taking as little as 5 or 10 units of insulin by the end of the summer, and I was sure he was crazy! After about ten days of eating macrobiotically, I was able to decrease my insulin dosage, dropping by 10-percent increments, from 65 units to 46 units. By June 20, it was down to 35 or 40 units, and some time in July, it went down to 30. Early in August, an experienced macrobiotic cook moved into the apartment where my father and I were staying, and after a short period of eating her cooking, my insulin suddenly took another leap downward.

In addition to the decrease in my insulin intake, I soon noticed a number of other changes. My acne diminished to a few small, dull bumps on my cheeks, and my complexion was brighter; my shoulders were suddenly straighter; and my energy calm and consistent from 8:00 A.M. to midnight. As the weeks became months, these changes were accentuated, and more deep-seated transformations became apparent as well. Most important, it became clear that one old, deeply ingrained assumption of mine was no longer true. This was the assumption that I would not live past the age of thirty-five. With the constant feeling of my vitality ebbing away, every year and every month, this was a constant background in my awareness and approach to life. Now my daily insulin dosage is down to about 15 units, my vitality is ever increasing, and I am enjoying every minute of it, since I know that all my dreams, all my potential will be realized. If I can change this much in a year, anybody else can change, too!

SIXTEEN

Macrobiotic
Home Remedies

Macrobiotics is concerned with keeping people well, through a wholesome diet, moderate exercise, and a balanced lifestyle. Although a balanced diet of whole foods is the best and safest path to good health, we must still be prepared for those times when the body may get out of balance. These imbalances may be due to past abuses, extreme environmental conditions, or other factors.

An essentially vegetarian macrobiotic diet, with the limited use of animal products, fish, and sweeteners, may be of benefit during recovery from certain serious illnesses. In addition, there are many traditional and natural home remedies that can be used as a part of home health care. The external application of compresses and plasters, as well as special combinations of foods and condiments, may be extremely helpful in certain cases.

The macrobiotic home remedies that follow are based on traditional medicines that have been used for thousands of years in many parts of the world to alleviate symptoms brought on by dietary and lifestyle imbalances.

If you have any doubts about the advisability of any of these home remedies, consult an experienced macrobiotic counselor before using them. People with serious illness are of course advised to seek appropriate medical, nutritional, and psychological care.

Macrobiotic counselors and others who already have some familiarity with macrobiotic home remedies will find the following list to be a useful reference. For each remedy, instructions for preparation follow a brief description of the item's purposes. If you are a newcomer to macrobiotics, and you are interested in using these home remedies, consult an experienced macrobiotic counselor first.

You will notice that almost all of these home remedies are derived from macrobiotic diet foods that are discussed elsewhere in this book. This is just one aspect of the Unifying Principle, that is, the interrelatedness of all things. The foods we eat do not merely satisfy hunger; they have a profound effect upon our health as well. Macrobiotics is the art of understanding these effects and using them to create balance and harmony.

Note that when preparing macrobiotic meals, it is important to use natural-material cookware (glass, ceramic, or earthenware) when preparing medicinal drinks.

BANCHA STEM TEA

Bancha stem tea is helpful in strengthening metabolism in the case of fatigue or illness. To prepare it, use 1 tablespoon of tea to 1 quart of water. Bring tea to a boil, reduce the flame, cover, and simmer for no more than five minutes. Use bancha stem tea after meals. In many cases, two to three cups a day may be used.

BARLEY-GREEN TEA

Barley green is the dried powder of young barley grass. It helps the body to burn fats and eliminate toxins arising from the use of animal foods. It also helps to cleanse the liver. To prepare, place 1–2 teaspoons of powder in a cup. Add hot water and drink. Consult an experienced macrobiotic counselor for advice regarding how long to use it.

BROWN RICE CREAM

Brown rice cream is especially helpful in cases in which digestion is impaired due to a debilitating illness. To prepare, wash brown rice and then dry-roast it evenly in a skillet until all the grains turn golden in color. Add three to six parts water and a little sea salt and pressure-cook for two hours. Squeeze the creamy portion of the cooked rice gruel through a clean cheesecloth. Serve the rice cream with a small amount of condiment such as umeboshi plum, gomashio, tekka, kelp, or kombu powder. Rice cream may be used two or more times a day, in whatever amount is desired.

BROWN RICE PLASTER

Brown rice plaster is used to reduce heat and swelling on an unopened boil or infection. To make the plaster, grind seven parts cooked brown rice with two parts raw leafy green vegetables (such as the outer leaves of cabbage, collards, or kale), and one part raw nori sea vegetable. Grind in a suribachi— the more the mixture is ground, the better. If it gets too sticky, add pure spring water. Apply paste to the affected area and cover with a clean cloth or towel. If the plaster heats up, remove it, clean the area with warm water, and repeat if desired.

BUCKWHEAT PLASTER

Buckwheat plaster helps to draw retained water or excess fluid from tissues through the skin. It can be used effectively to reduce swelling due to water retention. To prepare, mix buckwheat flour with enough hot water to form a stiff dough. Apply a half-inch layer to the affected area and hold it in place with a clean bandage or piece of cotton gauze. For either of the problems mentioned above, you may replace the plaster every four hours. A buckwheat plaster will usually reduce swelling considerably after only several applications, or at most two to three days.

BURDOCK TEA

Burdock tea is a tonic used for increasing overall vitality. To prepare, add a tablespoon of burdock root shavings to one cup of water. Bring to a boil, reduce flame, cover, and simmer for ten minutes.

DAIKON

Grated raw daikon is a digestive aid, especially when eaten with fatty, oily, or heavy foods, including animal products and fish. To prepare, grate a tablespoon of fresh daikon per person, and sprinkle with tamari soy sauce. Use raw red radish or raw turnip if daikon is not available.

DAIKON DRINKS

Three excellent drinks can be made using daikon radish. The first is helpful in reducing a fever by inducing perspiration. The second can be used as a diuretic, and the third helps to dissolve excess fat and mucus in the body. To make the first drink, mix a half cup of freshly grated daikon with a tablespoon of tamari soy sauce and one-quarter teaspoon of freshly grated ginger. Pour hot bancha tea over the mixture. Drink hot.

To make the second drink, squeeze 2 tablespoons of juice from grated daikon, using a clean cheesecloth. Add a pinch of sea salt and 6 tablespoons of water to the daikon juice, and boil. Use this mixture only once a day and never for more than three consecutive days. Do not drink the juice without first boiling it.

To make the third daikon drink, place 1 tablespoon of freshly grated daikon and 10 drops of tamari into a cup. Pour hot water over the mixture and drink. The best time to use this drink is just before sleeping. However, do not continue to use it for more than seven days, unless advised by an experienced macrobiotic counselor.

DANDELION ROOT TEA

Dandelion root tea helps tone and strengthen the heart and the small intestine. To prepare, mix 1 tablespoon of dried dandelion root into 1 quart of water and bring to a boil. Reduce the flame, cover, and simmer for ten minutes. Consult a macrobiotic counselor regarding the use of this tea.

DENTIE

Dentie has been used in Asia for years to prevent tooth and gum problems and to stop bleeding in nosebleeds and superficial cuts and abrasions. When used regularly in place of commercial toothpaste, dentie is effective in stopping bleeding of the gums, tightening teeth, and preventing decay. Dentie powder and paste can be purchased at health-food stores or made at home. To make dentie, bake a small eggplant, including the top, at 350°F until it is black. Let it cool before crushing it into a powder. Mix seven parts powder with three parts sea salt. Store in a covered dry container.

DRIED DAIKON LEAF SKIN WASH
OR HIP BATH

Dried daikon leaves are especially helpful in correcting skin problems and disorders of the female reproductive organs. They also work to draw excess oils and odors from the skin. Dry the leaves of several daikon radish plants in a shaded area until they turn brown and brittle. Use turnip leaves if daikon leaves are not available. The dried leaves may be stored in a covered dry container for up to a year.

To prepare, place between 20 and 30 leaves in 4–5 quarts of water. Bring mixture to a boil, reduce flame, cover, and simmer for fifteen minutes or until the water becomes brown. Stir in a handful of sea salt. Strain out the leaves, returning the liquid to the pot.

For skin problems, dip a clean piece of cotton or a cotton washcloth into the hot liquid, squeeze most of the hot liquid from it, and making sure it won't burn the skin, apply to the affected area. As the cloth cools, remove it and reapply until the skin is quite heated. For disorders of the female reproductive organs, pour the liquid into a hot bath (waist level). Cover your upper body with a towel and sit in the bath for about ten minutes or until perspiration begins. Arame can also be used for the bath. Following the bath, douche with warm bancha tea with the juice of half a lemon and a pinch of sea salt added to it. Repeat as needed for up to ten days.

GINGER COMPRESS

The ginger compress is used to stimulate circulation of the blood and lymph. When applied to the skin, it helps to loosen and dissolve stagnated

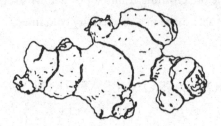

Figure 16.1   Ginger Root

toxic matter, cysts, and tumors. However, in the case of cancer illness, it should be used for a short time only (five minutes maximum) as a preparation for a taro potato or buckwheat plaster. *Note:* If used as an independent treatment, the ginger compress could potentially accelerate the growth of cancer, especially of yin types.

To prepare a ginger compress, grate a handful of ginger root and place it in a clean cheesecloth. (See Figure 16.1.) Squeeze the juice into a pot containing a gallon of hot (but not boiling) water. Do not boil the mixture. To use, dip a clean cotton towel into the ginger water and wring it out tightly, as illustrated in Figure 16.2. While it is still hot, place it on the affected area. Another (dry) towel can be placed on top of the ginger compress to reduce heat loss. Apply a fresh hot towel every five to seven minutes until the skin is quite heated.

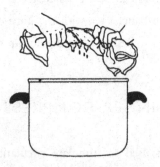

Figure 16.2   Ginger Compress

GINGER-SESAME OIL

Applied to the skin, ginger-sesame oil stimulates circulation by activating the function of the blood capillaries. It is also used to relieve aches and pains. To prepare it, mix the juice of freshly grated ginger with an equal amount of sesame oil. Apply it by dipping a piece of clean cotton gauze into the mixture and rub it briskly on the affected area.

GREEN TEA

Green tea helps dissolve and discharge animal fats and excess cholesterol from the body. To make this tea, place a half teaspoon of tea into a ceramic teapot. Pour 1 cup of boiling water over it and let it steep for three to five minutes. Strain and drink. Limit your use of green tea to one cup per day. This tea is not recommended for use by individuals with an overly yin condition or illness.

KOMBU TEA

Kombu tea helps to improve the quality of the blood and remineralize the body. To prepare it, place a three-inch strip of kombu sea vegetable in a quart of water. Bring it to a boil, reduce flame, cover, and simmer for ten minutes. Remove the kombu and serve the tea.

KUZU (KUDZU) TEA

Kuzu tea strengthens digestion, increases overall vitality, and reduces fatigue. To prepare it, dissolve a heaping teaspoon of kuzu in a cup of cold water and stir. Bring the mixture to a slight boil, reduce the flame, and simmer for about five minutes, stirring occasionally. The mixture is ready when it becomes transparent. Stir in a teaspoon of tamari soy sauce and drink it while it is still hot.

LOTUS ROOT PLASTER

Lotus root plaster helps draw stagnated mucus from the sinuses, nose, throat, and bronchi. To prepare, mix sixteen parts freshly grated lotus root with three parts whole-wheat pastry flour and one part freshly grated ginger. To apply, spread a half-inch layer on a piece of cotton gauze, and place the side with the lotus root directly on the affected area. Leave the plaster on for several hours or overnight. A ginger compress (page 225) can be applied before using the lotus root plaster to stimulate circulation and to loosen mucus in the affected area.

LOTUS ROOT TEA

Lotus root tea is especially helpful in relieving coughs and dissolving mucus in the lungs. To prepare it, squeeze the juice from a half cup of freshly grated lotus root into a pot with one cup of water. Simmer until the liquid thickens, add a pinch of sea salt, and drink it hot.

If fresh lotus root is unavailable, dried lotus root can be used instead. To make tea from the dried root, add 2 tablespoons of lotus root to 1 cup of water. Bring to a boil, reduce the flame, and simmer for fifteen minutes. Add a pinch of sea salt or a dash of tamari, and drink it hot.

MUSTARD PLASTER

Mustard plaster is used to stimulate circulation and to loosen stagnated materials from an affected area. To prepare a mustard plaster for an adult, add enough hot water to dry mustard powder to make a paste. Spread this mixture onto a paper towel, cover with another, and place this "sandwich" between two thick cotton towels. Apply it to the affected area and leave it on until the skin becomes quite warm. Remove and wash any remaining mustard from the skin with warm water.

SALT BANCHA TEA

Salt bancha tea is used to cleanse the body passages of stagnated matter. To prepare it, add about a half teaspoon of sea salt per cup of warm (body temperature) bancha tea. To cleanse the nasal passageways, inhale a small amount of the mixture through one nostril at a time, and expectorate rather than swallow any that reaches the mouth. Salt bancha tea can also be used as a mouthwash to soothe a sore throat, or as a douche to cleanse the vaginal region.

SALT PACK

Salt packs can be used to warm any part of the body and to relieve muscle stiffness, aches and pains, or eliminative problems where the use of heat is desired. To prepare a salt pack, roast sea salt in a dry skillet until it is hot. Use enough salt to cover the affected area with a layer a half-inch thick. Wrap the hot salt in a thick cotton pillowcase or towel. Place a folded towel on the affected area to prevent burns, and apply the salt pack. Replace the pack with another when it begins to cool.

SALT WATER

A pint of water with 2–4 tablespoons of sea salt in it can be used either cold or hot in various ways. Cold salt water is effective in soothing irritations caused by minor burns. To use, soak the burned area in a basin of cold salt water. Warm (body temperature) salt water is effective as an enema for relief of constipation or fat and mucus accumulation in the lower bowel. It may also be used as a douche to dissolve fat and mucus accumulations in the vagina.

SESAME OIL

Sesame oil is effective in relieving constipation. To use it for this purpose, mix 1–2 tablespoons of raw sesame oil with a quarter teaspoon each of freshly grated ginger and tamari soy sauce. Take this mixture on an empty stomach.

SHIITAKE MUSHROOM TEA

Shiitake mushroom tea acts as a mild relaxant to relieve overly tense muscles and nerves. It also helps dissolve excess animal fats. To prepare it, soak a dried shiitake mushroom in 1 cup of water for twenty minutes, then cut it into quarters. Add another cup of water and simmer for twenty minutes with a pinch of sea salt. Drink only a half cup at a time.

TAMARI BANCHA TEA

Tamari bancha tea helps neutralize an overly acid blood condition. To prepare, pour one cup of bancha twig tea into a teacup and stir in 2 teaspoons of tamari. Drink hot.

TARO POTATO (ALBI) PLASTER

Taro potato plaster has the effect of removing toxins from the body. It is especially effective in drawing the minerals that are often contained in tumors out through the skin. When used regularly in combination with the macrobiotic diet, taro plasters will help to gradually reduce the size of tumors.

Taro potatoes can be obtained at many supermarkets and from Chinese, Armenian, Portuguese, and Caribbean grocers. Taro are shaped like regular potatoes, with brown hair on them. (See Figure 16.3.) Buy relatively small potatoes for use in the plaster.

In many cases, it is best to apply a ginger compress (page 225) before using the taro plaster. To prepare the plaster, peel and grate enough potatoes to cover the area with a half-inch-thick layer. Add one part freshly grated ginger root for every nineteen parts grated potato. Apply a half-inch-thick layer of this mixture to a piece of clean cotton linen as shown in Figure 16.4. Place the side with the potato directly onto the affected area. Change every four hours. If desired, the plaster may be left on overnight without changing. If

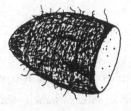

Figure 16.3   Taro Potato (Albi)

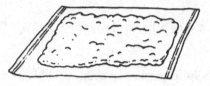

Figure 16.4   Taro Potato Plaster

the affected area becomes cold, replace the plaster with a hot ginger compress for three minutes before placing another plaster on the area. If the chill persists, use a salt pack (see page 229) to warm the area, but do not overheat.

If taro potatoes are not available in your area, you can purchase dried taro powder and make a plaster by adding pure spring water and ginger root to it. Or you can grate an ordinary potato and mix eight parts of it with eight parts crushed (use mortar and pestle to crush) raw leafy green vegetables such as the outer leaves of cabbage, collard greens, or kale, one part freshly grated ginger, and enough whole-wheat flour to make a paste. While not as effective as a taro plaster, this will still produce a beneficial result.

TOFU PLASTER

A tofu plaster is effective in drawing out a fever. To prepare it, squeeze the water out and mash the tofu. For every six parts of tofu, add one part freshly grated ginger and three parts whole-wheat pastry flour. Mix the ingredients together to make a paste and apply it directly to the skin. Change the plaster every two or three hours, or sooner if it becomes very hot.

UME EXTRACT

Ume extract is made from umeboshi plums. It is available at many health-foods store. To use it, pour hot water or bancha tea over a quarter teaspoon of the extract, and drink it hot.

UMEBOSHI PLUM

Umeboshi plums can be eaten fresh (pitted), dried and powdered, or baked. In any of these forms, umeboshi helps to normalize digestion. It is especially helpful in reducing stomach acidity and in relieving temporary intestinal ailments. To use, take a half or whole plum with a cup of bancha tea. Powdered umeboshi may be taken with either hot water or bancha tea. Place a tablespoon of powdered umeboshi plum in one cup of hot water or tea, and drink hot.

UME-SHO-BANCHA

Ume-sho-bancha strengthens the blood and overall condition through normalizing digestion. To prepare it, pour 1 cup of bancha tea over the meat of half an umeboshi plum and 1 teaspoon of tamari soy sauce. Stir and drink it hot.

A variation of the above can be made with ginger. Like ume-sho-bancha, this tea aids digestion and also stimulates circulation. Prepare as above, adding a quarter teaspoon of grated ginger juice to a cup of ume-sho-bancha.

UME-SHO-KUZU

Ume-sho-kuzu is especially helpful as a digestive aid. It also helps normalize and tone the intestines. Prepare kuzu drink according to the instructions given on page 227. Add half an umeboshi plum and 1 teaspoon of tamari soy sauce. One-eighth teaspoon of freshly grated ginger may also be added.

Epilogue

The natural world nourishes, supports, and sustains plant, animal, and human life. We, in turn, are to care for it with our utmost respect. A disregard for the natural world leads to plundering of the earth's resources and pollution of its atmosphere and water. A renewed commitment to the preservation of biological life and to the natural harmony between humans and nature can help us to resolve these and other problems that threaten our wholeness and our very survival.

At the very heart of the larger problems facing humanity is a fragmented and dualistic view of life. In the dualistic view, we see a hostile world: a struggle between good and bad, sickness and health, and love and hate. This fundamental division of thought underlies all of our economic, educational, scientific, and political institutions.

Macrobiotic theory is based on unity and wholeness, not division. The macrobiotic view recognizes that nature attempts to maintain harmony and balance. Health is seen as a natural result of balanced thinking, living, and eating. Societal health results when the members of an entire society live in harmony with the natural world.

The macrobiotic view that all life in the universe is a unified, orderly system controlled by definite natural laws makes each person acutely aware of his or her role as creator and shaper not only of individual lives, but also of the whole of life on earth. With the power that comes from this knowledge, we can consciously bring about the level of energy, variety of experience, and quality of life that we desire.

Macrobiotics states that eating natural, wholesome food is the first step toward better health and quality of life. While balanced exercise and activity strengthen and energize the body, self-reflection brings knowledge of our thoughts and desires, helping us to understand ourselves and the world around us. With these beginnings, the macrobiotic way can lead to a peaceful, cooperative, and loving world.

Appendix:
Nutritional Analysis of a Typical
Macrobiotic Daily Menu
Compared with the
U.S. DRIs

Throughout this book we have discussed the key nutrients supplied by the macrobiotic diet. In the chart that follows, this information is summarized and compared with the U.S. dietary reference intakes (DRIs) for adults. The results of the analysis show that the macrobiotic diet more than satisfies the DRIs for all the necessary nutrients.

The most important factor in ensuring that all the key nutrients are supplied every day by the macrobiotic diet is the use of a variety of the recommended foods, and the proper cooking of them. When eaten in the suggested proportion with one another (see Chapter 1), these foods supply enough high-quality nutrients to maintain excellent health and vitality.

Estimated Nutritional Analysis of a Typical Macrobiotic Menu*

The following menu is for one person for one day.

Food	Amount	Calories	GRAMS			MILLIGRAMS					IU	MILLIGRAMS			
MEASUREMENT UNITS			Protein	Fat	Carbohydrates	Calcium	Phosphorus	Iron	Sodium	Potassium	Vitamin A	Vitamin B₁ (thiamine)	Vitamin B₂ (riboflavin)	Vitamin B₃ (niacin)	Vitamin C
Breakfast															
Oatmeal	2 cups	260	10.0	2.0	46.0	44	232	3.0	344	292	0	0.38	0.10	0.4	0
Whole-wheat sourdough bread with apple butter	2 slices; 2 tablespoons	210	5.1	1.2	43.7	54	150	1.8	257	245	trace	0.18	0.06	1.6	trace
Bancha tea	1 cup	2	—	trace	0.4	—	—	trace	—	—	—	—	—	—	—
Lunch															
Cucumber sushi and tempeh-sauerkraut sushi	¼ recipe	420	17.8	6.2	65.4	61	177	12.1	497	246	800	0.41	0.34	6.9	25
Boiled salad with tofu dressing	1 serving	86	7.3	1.6	12.9	107	77	5.8	166	616	1,055	0.16	0.18	1.3	68
Bancha tea	1 cup	2	—	trace	0.4	—	—	trace	—	—	—	—	—	—	—
Snack															
Roasted almonds and sunflower seeds with raisins	½ cup	318	8.1	16.0	39.0	88	279	3.1	17	594	16	1.10	0.30	1.5	trace

Food	Amount	Grams				Milligrams					IU	Milligrams			
MEASUREMENT UNITS		Calories	Protein	Fat	Carbohydrates	Calcium	Phosphorus	Iron	Sodium	Potassium	Vitamin A	Vitamin B₁ (thiamine)	Vitamin B₂ (riboflavin)	Vitamin B₃ (niacin)	Vitamin C
Dinner															
Miso soup	1 bowl	59	3.0	0.7	7.7	148	96	6.9	349	205	83	0.50	0.70	0.4	22
Baked sole with rice	1 serving	396	21.5	9.5	70.4	66	378	2.8	361	525	140	0.25	0.11	6.6	trace
Grated daikon	¼ cup	5	0.3	—	1.0	9	6	0.2	150	195	3	—	—	—	10
Quickly boiled watercress and carrots with umeboshi-scallion dressing	1 serving	81	3.3	2.6	8.5	264	82	1.8	165	350	12,662	0.06	0.02	1.0	80
Couscous cake with pear sauce	1 serving	287	2.6	0.4	65.7	18	62	1.8	254	398	30	0.03	0.04	0.6	31
Grain coffee	1 cup	—	—	—	—	—	—	—	—	—	—	—	—	—	—
TOTALS		2,126	79.0	40.2	361.1	859	1,539	39.3	2,560	3,666	14,789	3.07	1.85	20.3	236

Note: A dash signifies a lack of reliable data for a constituent believed to be present in a measurable amount.

Source: *Estimated nutritional content of this macrobiotic menu is based on USDA Composition of Foods Handbook No. 8.

Summary—Typical Macrobiotic Menu Totals Compared with the U.S. DRIs

Food	Amount	Grams				Milligrams					Vitamin A	Milligrams			
MEASUREMENT UNITS		Calories	Protein	Fat	Carbohydrates	Calcium	Phosphorus	Iron	Sodium₃	Potassium	IU	Vitamin B₁ (thiamine)	Vitamin B₂ (riboflavin)	Vitamin B₃ (niacin)	Vitamin C
Macrobiotic menu totals[1]	All	2,126	79.0	40.2	361.1	859	1,539	39.3	2,560	3,666	14,789	3.07	1.85	20.3	236
U.S. DRIs—males[2]	Ages 19–50	1,800–2,500	54–75	—	—	1,000	700	8	—	—	3,000	1.20	1.30	16.0	90
U.S. DRIs—females[2]	Ages 19–50	1,200–1,600	36–48	—	—	1,000	700	18	—	—	2,330	1.10	1.10	14.0	75

Note: A dash signifies a lack of reliable data for a constituent believed to be present in a measurable amount.

1. Estimated nutritional content of this macrobiotic menu is based on *USDA Composition of Foods Handbook No. 8.*

2. The figures for DRIs were established by the Food and Nutrition Board, Institute of Medicine, National Institutes, 2001.

3. There is no established DRI for sodium, but average daily sodium intake among American adults is 6,000–18,000 milligrams, which most experts agree is far higher than it should be.

Glossary

The following glossary describes macrobiotic foods, cooking methods, kitchen equipment, and ideas that may not be familiar to you. Words that have particular application to the relationship between diet and health are also included.

Acupressure. A healing art based on stimulating and balancing the flow of electromagnetic energy through the meridians of the body. Acupressure utilizes finger and hand pressure on acupuncture points of the body.

Acupuncture. A Far Eastern medical technique used to reestablish balance and relieve pain by releasing blockages of energy. Acupuncture uses needles or *moxa* (a substance that is burned) placed on or in specific points along the meridians.

Additives, chemical. Any of the various artificial flavorings, coloring agents, or preservatives, not naturally found in foods, that are used in refining and processing. More than 3,000 chemical additives have been approved by the U.S. Food and Drug Administration.

Adzuki beans. Small, dark-red beans. Especially good when cooked with kombu. This bean may also be referred to as *aduki* or *azuki*.

Agar-agar.   A white gelatinous substance derived from a sea vegetable. Agar-agar is used in making aspics and kanten. *See also* Kanten.

Albi.   *See* Taro.

Amasake (rice milk).   A sweetener or refreshing drink made from sweet rice and koji starter that is allowed to ferment into a thick liquid. Hot amasake is a delicious beverage on cold autumn or winter nights.

Arame.   A dark-brown, spaghettilike sea vegetable similar to hijiki. Rich in iron, calcium, and other minerals, arame is often used as a side dish.

Arrowroot.   A starch flour processed from the root of an American native plant. It is used as a thickening agent, similar to cornstarch or kuzu, for making sauces, stews, and desserts.

Azuki.   *See* Adzuki beans.

Bancha tea.   Correctly named *kukicha*, bancha consists of the twigs and leaves from mature Japanese tea bushes. Bancha aids digestion, is high in calcium, and contains no chemical dyes. It makes an excellent breakfast or after-dinner beverage.

Barley, pearl.   A strain of barley native to China, pearl barley grows well in cold climates. It is good in stews and soups, or cooked with other grains. Pearl barley helps the body to eliminate animal fats.

Barley malt.   A thick, dark-brown sweetener made from barley. Pure (100 percent) barley malt is used in making desserts, sweet and sour sauces, and in a variety of medicinal drinks.

Beans.   See Adzuki beans; Japanese black beans.

Beefsteak plant.   *See* Shiso.

Black sesame seeds.   Small black seeds used occasionally as a garnish or to make black gomashio, a condiment. These seeds are different from the usual white or tan variety.

Black soybeans.   *See* Japanese black beans.

Bok choy.   A leafy, green vegetable with thick white stems that resemble stalks. Bok choy is used mostly in summer cooking. It is sometimes called *pok choy.*

Bread, sprouted-wheat.   A whole-grain bread made from soaked wheat that is sprouted and baked. Sprouted-wheat bread does not contain flour, salt, or oil, and is very sweet and moist.

Brown rice.   Unpolished rice with only its tough outer husk removed. It comes in three main varieties: short, medium, and long grain. Short-grain brown rice contains the best balance of minerals, protein, and carbohydrates, but the other types may also be used on occasion. *See also* Sweet brown rice.

Brown rice miso.   *See* Genmai miso.

Brown rice vinegar.   A very mild and delicate vinegar made from fermented brown rice or sweet brown rice. Brown rice vinegar is not as acid-forming in the body as apple cider vinegar.

Buckwheat.   A cereal plant native to Siberia, buckwheat has been a staple food in many European countries for several centuries. It is frequently eaten in the form of kasha, whole groats, or soba noodles.

Burdock.   A hardy plant that grows wild throughout the United States. The long, dark burdock root is delicious in soups, stews, and sea vegetable dishes, or sautéed with carrots. It is highly valued in macrobiotic cooking for its strengthening qualities. The Japanese name is *gobo*.

Carbohydrates, complex.   Those starches, known chemically as polysaccharides, which provide the body with a high proportion of usable energy over a period of several hours. Complex carbohydrates are the major component of the macrobiotic diet. A source of energy, they are supplied primarily by whole grains, vegetables, and beans.

Chemical additives.   See Additives, chemical.

Chinese cabbage.   A large, leafy vegetable with pale-green tops and thick white stems. Sometimes called *nappa,* this juicy, slightly sweet vegetable is good in soups and stews, vegetable dishes, and pickled.

Cholesterol.   A compound manufactured in the human body, important in the structure of membranes and the formation of certain hormones. Cholesterol is also a constituent of all animal products. When consumed in excess in the diet, cholesterol increases the risk of gallstones, heart disease, cancer, and other health problems.

Complex carbohydrates.   See Carbohydrates, complex.

Condition.   An individual's present state of health, rather than his or her state of health at birth, or *constitution.*

Constitution.   An individual's characteristics, determined before birth by the health and vitality of his or her parents, grandparents, and other ancestors. *See also* Condition.

Couscous.   A partially refined and quick-cooking cracked wheat that has a flavor similar to cream of wheat.

Daikon.   A long, white radish. Besides making a delicious side dish, daikon helps dissolve stagnant fat and mucous deposits that have accumulated in the body. Freshly grated raw daikon is especially helpful in the digestion of oily foods.

Daikon, dried.   Daikon sold in dried and shredded form. Dried daikon is especially good cooked with kombu and seasoned with tamari soy sauce. Soaking dried daikon before use brings out its natural sweetness.

Discharge. The body's elimination of stored mucus, fat, and toxins through a variety of means, including urination, defecation, perspiration, coughing, boils, cysts, and tumors.

Do-in. A form of Oriental exercise and self-massage that works to harmonize and balance the electromagnetic energy flowing through the meridians.

Dulse. A reddish-purple sea vegetable used in soups, salads, and vegetable dishes. Dulse is high in protein, iron, vitamin A, iodine, and phosphorus. Most of the dulse sold in America comes from Canada, Maine, and Massachusetts.

Electromagnetic energy. Energy that flows through all things, including the human body. Electromagnetic energy is generated by the earth's rotation and orbit.

Fermentation. The action of certain bacteria or enzymes, changing the chemical composition of foods and making them easier to digest. Fermented foods on the macrobiotic diet include sauerkraut, pickles, sourdough breads, and some soyfoods.

Fiber. The indigestible portion of whole foods; particularly, the bran of whole grains and the outer skin of legumes, vegetables, and fruits. Fiber facilitates the passage of waste through the intestines. Foods that are refined, processed, or peeled are low in fiber.

Fu. A dried wheat-gluten product. Available in thin sheets or thick round cakes, fu is a satisfying high-protein food used in soups, stews, and vegetable dishes.

Genmai miso. Miso made from soybeans, brown rice, and sea salt, fermented for approximately twelve months. Used in making soups and seasoning vegetable dishes. Also called *brown rice miso.*

Ginger. A spicy, pungent, golden-colored root, used as a garnish or seasoning in cooking and for various beverages. Also used in making external home remedies such as the ginger compress.

Ginger compress. A hot compress, made from the juice of ginger root and water, which stimulates circulation and dissolves stagnation in the part of the body to which it is applied.

Gluten, wheat. The sticky substance that remains after the bran has been kneaded and rinsed from whole-wheat flour. Gluten is used to make seitan and fu.

Gobo. *See* Burdock.

Gomashio. Also known as *sesame salt.* Gomashio is a table condiment made from roasted, ground sesame seeds and sea salt. It is good sprinkled on brown rice and other whole grains.

Goma wakame powder.   A condiment made from roasted and crushed wakame and sesame seeds. Rich in minerals and other essential nutrients, goma wakame powder can be used like gomashio.

Gomoku rice.   A hearty dish traditionally made from varied combinations of four whole grains and one type of bean. Gomoku is especially good during the autumn and winter months.

Grain coffee.   A nonstimulating, caffeine-free coffee substitute made from roasted grains, beans, and roots. Ingredients are combined in different ways to create a variety of different flavors. Used like instant coffee.

Green nori flakes.   A sea vegetable condiment made from a certain type of nori, different from the packaged variety. The flakes are rich in iron, calcium, and vitamin A. They can be sprinkled on whole grains, vegetables, salads, and other dishes.

Hatcho miso.   Miso made from soybeans and sea salt and fermented for a minimum of two years. It has a mild salt taste and may be used from time to time in making soup stocks and condiments, and for seasoning vegetable dishes. This dark, rich miso is especially good in cold weather.

Hijiki.   A dark-brown sea vegetable that turns black when dried. It has a spaghetti-like consistency, a stronger taste than arame, and is very high in calcium and protein. The hijiki sold in the United States is imported from Japan or harvested off the coast of Maine.

Hokkaido pumpkin.   There are two varieties of Hokkaido pumpkin. One has a deep orange color and the other has a light-green skin similar to Hubbard squash. Both varieties are very sweet and have a tough outer skin.

Hydrogenation.   A process by which vegetable oils are made more saturated, causing them to become denser and more solid.

Japanese black beans.   A special type of soybean grown in Japan. They can be used to alleviate problems of the reproductive organs. In cooking, these black beans are used in soups and side dishes.

Kampyo.   Dried gourd strips that are first soaked and then used to bind vegetable rolls. The kampyo can be eaten along with the vegetable rolls.

Kanten.   A jelled dessert made from agar-agar. It can include seasonal fruits such as melon, apples, berries, peaches, and pears, or amasake, adzuki beans, and other foods. Usually served chilled, it is a refreshing alternative to conventional gelatin.

Kasha.   Buckwheat groats that are roasted prior to boiling. Kasha is a traditional Eastern European and Russian food.

Kayu. Cereal grain cooked with five to ten times as much water as grain for a long period of time. Kayu is ready when it is soft and creamy.

Kelp. A large family of sea vegetables that grow profusely off both coasts of the United States. Kelp is widely available at natural foods stores, packaged whole, granulated, or powdered. It is an excellent source of minerals, including iodine.

Kinpura. Sautéed root vegetables cut into matchsticks, usually burdock or burdock and carrots seasoned with tamari soy sauce. This hearty dish is warming and vitalizing, making it ideal for autumn and winter use.

Koji. A grain, usually semi-polished or polished rice, inoculated with bacteria and used to begin the fermentation process in a variety of foods, including miso, amasake, tamari, natto, and sake.

Kokkoh. A porridge especially for babies, made from brown rice, sweet brown rice, adzuki beans, sesame seeds, and kombu. A little yinnie (rice) syrup or barley malt may be used to sweeten it.

Kombu. A wide, thick, dark-green sea vegetable that is rich in minerals. Kombu is often cooked with beans and vegetables. A single piece may be reused several times to flavor soup stocks.

Konnyaku. A gelatinous mold made in Japan from wild mountain potatoes. There are several varieties; all must be boiled and rinsed to remove their strong, bitter taste before they are added to other dishes. Used in sea vegetable and nishime dishes.

Kudzu. *See* Kuzu.

Kukicha. *See* Bancha tea.

Kuzu. A white starch made from the root of the wild kuzu plant. In this country, the plant densely populates the southern states, where it is called *kudzu*. It is used in making soups, sauces, desserts, and medicinal beverages.

Lotus. The root and seeds of a water lily that is brown-skinned with a hollow, chambered, off-white inside. Lotus is especially good for the sinuses and lungs. The seeds are used in grain, bean, and sea vegetable dishes.

Macrobiotics. An approach to balanced living, based on a balanced diet, moderate exercise, harmony with the environment, and an understanding of the philosophic principles of yin and yang. George Ohsawa was the first to recognize how these traditional concepts could be applied to modern living.

Meridian. In Oriental medicine, a pathway through which electromagnetic energy flows in the body. The healing arts acupuncture, shiatzu, and *do-in,* along with the martial arts, strive to reestablish harmony of the energy flow through the many meridians of the body.

Millet. A small yellow grain that comes in many varieties, with pearled millet being the most common. Millet is used in soups, vegetable dishes, casseroles, and as a cereal.

Mirin. A cooking wine made from whole-grain sweet rice. Be careful when purchasing mirin, as many varieties on the market have been processed with refined grain and additives.

Miso. A protein-rich fermented soybean paste made from ingredients such as soybeans, barley, and brown or white rice. Miso is used in soup stocks and as a seasoning. When consumed on a regular basis, it aids circulation and digestion. Mugi miso is usually best for daily use, but other varieties may be used occasionally. Quick or short-term misos, which are fermented for several weeks, are less suitable for frequent use; their salt content is higher than that of the longer-term varieties such as mugi and hatcho miso. *See also* Genmai miso; Hatcho miso; Mugi miso; Natto miso; Onazaki miso; Red miso; White miso; Yellow miso.

Miso, puréed. Miso that has been reduced to a smooth, creamy texture that will allow it to blend easily with other ingredients. To purée miso, place it in a bowl or suribachi and add enough water or broth to make a smooth paste. Blend with a wooden pestle or spoon.

Mochi. A heavy rice cake or dumpling made from cooked, pounded sweet brown rice. Mochi is especially good for lactating mothers, as it promotes the production of breast milk. Mochi can be prepared at home or purchased ready-made; it makes an excellent snack.

Mugicha. A tea made from roasted unhulled barley and water. Mugicha may be served hot or as a refreshing chilled beverage in the summer.

Mucus. Secretion of mucous membranes, normally serving to protect and lubricate many parts of the body. Illness, environmental pollution, smoking, and the consumption of excess fats, sugar, and flour products can stimulate the overproduction of mucus and clog body passageways, preventing the body from expelling harmful substances.

Mugi miso. A miso made from barley, soybeans, and sea salt, fermented for about eighteen to twenty-four months. This flavorful miso can be used on a daily basis year-round to make soup stocks, condiments, and pickles, and to season vegetable or bean dishes. Mugi miso is generally suitable for use by individuals with serious illness.

Mu tea. Tea made from a blend of traditional, non-stimulating herbs. A warming and strengthening beverage, mu tea is especially beneficial for the female reproductive organs. Two popular varieties of mu tea are #9 and #16.

Nappa. *See* Chinese cabbage.

Natto. Soybeans that have been cooked, mixed with beneficial enzymes, and allowed to ferment for twenty-four hours. Natto is high in easy-to-digest protein and vitamin B_{12}.

Natto miso. A condiment made from soybeans, barley, kombu, and ginger; not actually a miso.

Natural. Term used to describe foods that are not processed or treated with artificial additives or preservatives. Some natural foods are partially refined using traditional methods.

Nigari. A coagulant made from sea salt, used in making tofu.

Nishime. A method of cooking in which different combinations of vegetables, sea vegetables, or soybean products are slow-cooked with a small amount of water and tamari soy sauce. Also referred to as *waterless cooking*.

Nori. Thin black or dark-purple sheets of dried sea vegetable. Nori is often roasted over a flame until it turns green. It is used as a garnish, wrapped around rice balls in making sushi, or cooked with tamari soy sauce as a condiment. It is rich in vitamins and minerals. It is sometimes called *laver*.

Oden. A dish in which root vegetables, sea vegetables, soybean products, and sometimes fish are simmered together for a long time. Many combinations of ingredients are used in making this excellent winter stew.

Ohagi. Glutenous patties made from cooked, pounded sweet rice rolled in or coated with roasted and ground sesame seeds, roasted ground nuts, puréed adzuki beans and raisins, etc. Frequently eaten as a dessert.

Oil, refined. Salad or cooking oil that has been chemically extracted and processed to maximize yield and extend shelf life. Refining strips an oil of its color, flavor, and aroma, and reduces its nutritive value.

Oil, unrefined. Pressed and/or solvent-extracted vegetable oil that retains the original color, flavor, aroma, and nutritional value of the natural substance.

Onazaki miso. A miso made from white rice, soybeans, and sea salt. Lighter in color than mugi, hatcho, and genmai miso, and slightly saltier, onazaki miso has a rich flavor. It is used occasionally in making soup stocks and for seasoning vegetable dishes.

Organic. Term used to describe food that is grown and harvested without the use of synthetically compounded chemical fertilizers, pesticides, herbicides, and fungicides.

Pearl barley. *See* Barley, pearl.

Physiognomy. The art of judging an individual's state of health by viewing his or her facial and bodily characteristics.

Pok choy. *See* Bok choy.

Polyunsaturated. Term used to describe the molecular structure of the fats that are present in vegetable oils and other whole foods, including fish. While polyunsaturates are more healthful than saturated fats, overconsumption may lead to elevated fatty acid (triglyceride) levels in the bloodstream.

Pressed salad. Very thinly sliced or shredded fresh vegetables, combined with a pickling agent such as sea salt, umeboshi, brown rice vinegar, or tamari soy sauce, and placed in a pickle press. In the pickling process, many of the enzymes and vitamins are retained while the vegetables become easier to digest.

Red miso. A salty-tasting short-term fermented miso, made from soybeans and sea salt. Suitable for occasional use by individuals who are in good health. Also called *aka miso.*

Rice. *See* Brown rice; Gomoku rice; Sweet Brown rice; Wild rice.

Rice balls. Rice shaped into balls or triangles, usually with a piece of umeboshi in the center, and wrapped in toasted nori or shiso leaves to completely cover. For variety, different ingredients may be used as filling or for a coating. Rice balls are good for snacks, lunches, picnics, and traveling.

Rice milk. *See* Amasake.

Rice syrup. *See* Yinnie syrup.

Sake. Japanese rice wine containing about 15 percent alcohol, often used in cooking.

Sake lees. Fermented residue from making sake (rice wine), used occasionally as a seasoning in soups, stews, vegetable dishes, and pickles. Sake lees is especially good for use in winter, as it helps to generate body heat.

Sanpaku. A Japanese term meaning "three whites." In Oriental medicine, sanpaku describes a condition of the eyes in which the iris is generally turned upward so that white is visible beneath. This condition may be related to poor diet, and may also be a sign of ill health or misfortune.

Saturated. Term used to describe the molecular structure of most of the fats found in red meats, dairy products, and other animal foods. An excess of these in the diet contributes to heart disease and other illnesses.

Sea salt. Salt obtained from evaporated seawater, as opposed to rock salt mined from inland beds. Sea salt is either sun-baked or kiln-baked. High in trace minerals, it contains no sugar or chemical additives.

Sea vegetable. Any of a variety of marine plants used as food. Sea vegetables are a prime source of vitamins, minerals, and trace elements in the macrobiotic diet.

Seitan. Wheat gluten cooked in tamari soy sauce, kombu, and water. Seitan can be made at home or purchased ready-made at many natural foods stores. It is high in protein and has a chewy texture, making it an ideal meat substitute.

Sesame butter. A nut butter obtained by roasting and grinding brown sesame seeds until smooth and creamy. It is used like peanut butter or in salad dressings and sauces.

Shiatzu. A form of Oriental massage that releases blockages of electromagnetic energy and harmonizes energy flow through the meridians of the body.

Shiitake. A type of mushroom originally imported dried from Japan and now available freshly grown in many parts of the United States. Either type can be used to flavor soup stocks or vegetable dishes, and dried shiitake can also be used in medicinal preparations. These mushrooms help the body to discharge excess animal fats.

Shio kombu. Pieces of kombu cooked for a long time in tamari soy sauce and used sparingly as a condiment. Shio kombu has a strong salty taste.

Shio nori. Pieces of nori cooked for a long time in tamari soy sauce and water. Used occasionally as a condiment, shio nori makes a particularly tasty relish.

Shiso. A red, pickled leaf. The plant is known in English as the *beefsteak plant*. Shiso leaves are used to color umeboshi plums and as a condiment. Sometimes spelled *chiso*.

Shoyu. *See* Tamari and tamari soy sauce.

Simple sugar. A source of quick but short-lasting energy. Simple sugars include sucrose (table sugar), fructose, glucose (dextrose), and lactose (milk sugar). Up to 50 percent of the carbohydrates consumed in the average modern diet are simple sugars. *See also* Carbohydrates, complex.

Soba. Noodles made from buckwheat flour or a combination of buckwheat and whole-wheat flour. Soba can be served in broth, in salads, or with vegetables. In the summer, soba noodles are good chilled.

Somen. Very thin white or whole-wheat Japanese noodles. Thinner than soba and other whole-grain noodles, somen are often served during the summer.

Soy sauce. *See* Tamari and tamari soy sauce.

Sprouted-wheat bread. *See* Bread, sprouted-wheat.

Suribachi. A special serrated, glazed clay bowl. Used with a pestle, called a surikogi, for grinding and puréeing foods. An essential item in the macrobiotic kitchen, the suribachi can be used in a variety of ways to make condiments, spreads, dressings, baby foods, nut butters, and medicinal preparations.

Surikogi. A wooden pestle that is used with a suribachi. Used to make gomashio, sea vegetable powders, and other condiments, and to mash foods to obtain a creamy consistency.

Sushi. Rice rolled with vegetables, fish, or pickles, wrapped in nori, and sliced in rounds. Sushi is becoming increasingly popular throughout the United States. The most healthful sushi is made with brown rice and other natural ingredients.

Sushi mat. Very thin strips of bamboo that are fastened together with cotton thread so that they can be rolled tightly yet allow air to pass through freely. These mats are used in rolling sushi, and also to cover freshly cooked foods or leftovers.

Sweet brown rice. A sweeter-tasting, more glutenous variety of brown rice. Sweet brown rice is used in mochi, ohagi, dumplings, baby foods, vinegar, and amasake. It is often used in cooking for festive occasions.

Tahini. A nut butter obtained by grinding hulled white sesame seeds until smooth and creamy. It is used like sesame butter.

Takuan. Daikon that is pickled in rice bran and sea salt. It is named after the Buddhist priest who invented this particular pickling method. Sometimes spelled *takuwan*.

Tamari and tamari soy sauce. Tamari soy sauce is traditional, naturally made soy sauce, as distinguished from chemically processed varieties. Original or "real" tamari is the liquid poured off during the process of making hatcho miso. The best-quality tamari soy sauce is naturally fermented for more than a year and is made from whole soybeans, wheat, and sea salt. Tamari soy sauce is sometimes referred to as *shoyu*.

Taro. A type of potato with a thick, dark-brown, hairy skin. It is eaten as a vegetable or used in the preparation of plasters for medicinal purposes. Also called *albi*.

Tekka. A condiment made from hatcho miso, sesame oil, burdock, lotus root, carrot, and ginger root. Tekka is sautéed over a low flame for several hours. It is dark brown in color and very rich in iron.

Tempeh. A traditional soyfood, made from split soybeans, water, and beneficial bacteria, and allowed to ferment for several hours. Tempeh is eaten in Indonesia and Sri Lanka as a staple food. Rich in easy-to-digest protein and Vitamin B_{12}, tempeh is available prepackaged in some natural foods stores.

Tempura. A method of cooking in which seasonal vegetables and fish or seafood are coated with batter and deep-fried in unrefined oil. Tempura is often served with soup and pickles.

Tofu.   Soybean curd, made from soybeans and nigari. Tofu is a protein-rich soyfood used in soups, vegetable dishes, dressings, and so on. *See also* Tofu, dried.

Tofu, dried.   Tofu that has been naturally dehydrated by freezing. Used in soups, stews, and vegetable and sea vegetable dishes, dried tofu contains less fat than regular tofu. *See also* Tofu.

Toxin.   A poisonous compound of animal or vegetable origin that stimulates the production of antibodies.

Udon.   Japanese-style noodles made from wheat, whole-wheat, or whole-wheat and unbleached white flour. Udon have a lighter flavor than soba (buckwheat) noodles and can be used the same way.

Umeboshi.   Salty, pickled plums that stimulate the appetite and digestion, and aid in maintaining an alkaline blood quality. Shiso leaves impart a reddish color and natural flavoring to the plums during pickling. Umeboshi can be used whole or in the form of a paste.

Umeboshi vinegar.   A salty, sour vinegar made from umeboshi plums. Diluted with water, it is used in sweet and sour sauces, salads, salad dressings, and so on.

Unifying Principle.   The principle of yin and yang, the philosophical foundation of macrobiotics. The Unifying Principle states that everything in the universe is constantly changing and that antagonistic forces complement one another. An understanding of this principle promotes harmony of body and mind and helps individuals to achieve balance with the natural world. *See also* Yang; Yin.

Unsaturated.   *See* Polyunsaturated.

Wakame.   A long, thin, green sea vegetable used in making a variety of dishes. High in protein, iron, and magnesium, wakame has a sweet taste and delicate texture. It is especially good in miso soup.

Wasabi.   A light-green Japanese horseradish that is used in sushi or traditionally with raw fish (sashimi). Wasabi is a very hot spice.

Wheat gluten.   *See* Gluten, wheat.

Wheatberries.   The grains of whole wheat are often called wheatberries. They are used to make whole-wheat flours and noodles. They can also be soaked and pressure-cooked with brown rice or other whole grains.

White miso.   A sweet-tasting short-term fermented miso made from white rice, soybeans, and sea salt. Used in making soup stocks and sometimes in vegetable dishes. Suitable for occasional use by individuals who are in good health. Also called *shiro miso*.

Whole foods. The edible portions of foods as they come from nature, unprocessed, nutritionally complete, and without chemical additives. Whole foods are not refined at all.

Wild rice. A wild grass that grows in water and is harvested by hand. Eaten traditionally by native Americans in Minnesota and other areas. These long, dark, thin grains are available at many natural foods stores.

Yang. In macrobiotics, energy or movement that has a centripetal or inward direction. One of the two antagonistic yet complementary forces that together describe all phenomena, yang is traditionally symbolized by an upward-facing triangle (△). *See also* Unifying Principle; Yin.

Yellow miso. A short-term fermented miso made from white rice, soybeans, and sea salt. This miso has a salty but very mellow flavor and is used in making soups, sauces, and vegetable dishes. It is suitable for occasional use by individuals who are in good health.

Yin. In macrobiotics, energy or movement that has a centrifugal or outward direction and results in expansion. One of the two antagonistic yet complementary forces that together describe all phenomena, yin is traditionally symbolized by an inverted triangle (▽). *See also* Unifying Principle; Yang.

Yinnie syrup. A sweet, thick syrup made from brown rice and barley that is used in dessert cooking. This complex carbohydrate sweetener is preferable to simple sugars such as honey, maple syrup, and molasses, because the simple sugars are metabolized too quickly. Also called *rice syrup*.

Yu-dofu. A simmered tofu and vegetable dish served in a seasoned broth. Yu-dofu is popular throughout Japan and is ideal for autumn and winter evening meals. It may be served with a variety of dips, sauces, and garnishes.

Bibliographical Notes

The inset "Denmark's 'Macrobiotic Experiment'" on page 16 is from Mikkel Hindhede, "The Effects of Food Restriction During War on Mortality in Copenhagen," *Journal of the American Medical Association* 74 (1920): 381–382.

The inset "The Sweet Life of a Sugar Junkie" on page 21 is from *Sugar Blues* (Warner Books, 1975) © William Dufty. Used by permission.

The inset "A Vegetarian Baseball Team" on page 29 is from Irving Wallace, David Wallechinsky, and Amy Wallace, "Significa" *Parade Magazine* (April 1984). Used by permission.

The inset "Dirk Benedict's Battle" on page 48 is adapted from a story reported by Lois Armstrong in *People* (10 October 1983) © Time Inc. Used by permission.

The inset "Up from Hypoglycemia—A Case History" on page 64 is adapted from an article by Diane Sacolick in *MacroMuse Magazine,* issue 14 © 1984. Used by permission.

The inset "Beating Diabetes: Larry Bogoslaw's Story" on page 218 is by John Mann. Used by permission of Larry Bogoslaw and the author.

Classes and Further Information

Further information on implementing a natural foods diet can be obtained from the Kushi Institute, the world's leading macrobiotic educational center. Established in 1978 by Michio and Aveline Kushi, the Kushi Institute offers a variety of programs, including health recovery, professional training, and classes in macrobiotic cooking and shiatzu, among other natural healing fields. To find out about classes and seminars, obtain more recipes, shop on-line for mactobiotic foods, or to get the Kushi Institute newsletter, contact the Kushi Institute at the address below or visit them online.

Kushi Institute
PO Box 7
Becket, MA 01223
www.kushiinstitute.org

Index